Bonnie Prudden's

QUICK

Rx

FOR FITNESS

Photographs by Joel Librizzi

PUBLISHERS

Grosset & Dunlap

NEW YORK

A National General Company

TO MARGARET McSWIGGIN

HOW TO USE THIS BOOK

Just as there are specific medicines for particular conditions, there are specific exercises for particular problems. **All** exercises will improve circulation, endurance and general tone. **Some exercises are better than others** for improving such specifics as backache, a protruding abdomen or just being out of breath.

You know what your problem is. Locate it alphabetically in the TABLE OF CONTENTS. If you have only one problem, don't stop there. Add from the section on **Exercise Programs,** one that suits your level of fitness, and raise that level.

The heavy black numbers denote the more essential exercises for each particular problem; lighter numbers refer to exercises that are also helpful, but may be omitted if occasionally you are short of time.

The **musts** in the book are the tests and measurements at the very start . . . **and they are musts.** Since **you** will have to be responsible for your own program, you will need the tests to prove your own improvement to yourself. Just as the doctor uses laboratory tests that tell him yes, the hemoglobin is up or the eosinophile count is down, you will test, weigh and measure. Keep track of what happens . . . not only to your muscles and your clothing size, **but to the way you feel generally . . . and especially emotionally.**

Any doctor can give you a prescription for medicine, but **you** have to take it. Devote at least ten minutes a day (more if you want faster results) to your exercise prescription and grow stronger, more attractive, and feel younger. THEN GO OUT AND ENJOY IT.

CONTENTS

HANDS   page 90
Arthritis; Poor dexterity; Tension; Weak wrists.

HEART   page 20
Diet; Heart disease; Sudden activity; Inactivity.

HEEL CORDS (soleus)   page 86
Sport preparation; Tightness and inflexibility.

HIPS   page 68
Heaviness; Thinness; Fibrositis.

ISOMETRIC CONTRACTION   page 118

JUMP ROPE   page 132

KNEES   page 77
Aging; Contact sports; Inflexibility; Injury;
Weakness.

LEGS :   page 74
Arteriosclerosis; Cramps; Fat; Inflexibility; Ten-
sion; Thinness; Under-exercise; Varicose veins;
Weakness.

MEASUREMENTS   page 17
Charting improvement; How to measure; Menstrual periods; Muscle vs. fat; Weight and size.

MIDRIFF AND WAISTLINE   page 64
Fat and inflexibility.

NECK   page 46
Muscle spasm; Pain; Stress and tension.

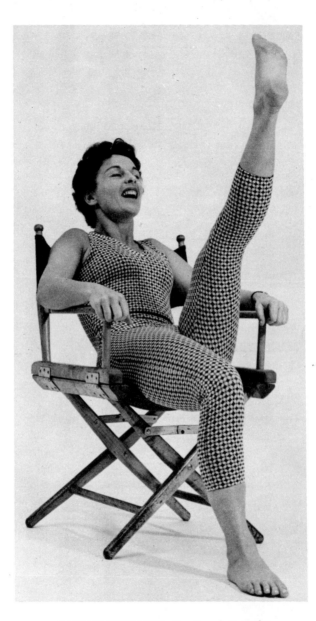

BONNIE PRUDDEN, *directing photography,*
throws herself into the job.

MINIMUM MUSCULAR FITNESS TEST

No matter what shape you are in today and no matter what you intend to do about it, your first step should be to determine exactly where you stand right now. You should know both how bad **and** how good you are, what needs fixing at once, and what you can forget about for the time being. Some problems will take care of themselves once you have corrected others.

Start by giving yourself (and anyone else you are interested in) the Kraus-Weber Test for Minimum Muscular Fitness (page **11**). It tests those key posture muscles needed for just plain everyday living, your back and your abdominals. It tests for weakness, which everybody understands, and for flexibility—which almost nobody understands. **Strength plus flexibility, in the proper timing and intensity, yield coordination.** That's why you will find so many exercises for the improvement of flexibility in this book.

If you are a tense sort of person, a driving person, and especially bright and busy, beware of inflexibility. Although everyone has some weakness, it is almost better to lack strength than to lack flexibility. Weakness can be corrected with far less effort in far less time.

In this country 80% of all the backaches are caused by either weakness or inflexibility, or by an unholy alliance between the two of them, not by "ruptured discs" or "a pinched nerve." (The term "sacroilliac" concerns an area, not a condition.) Although disc and nerve problems exist, probably less than 20% of America's backaches are caused by these and other forms of pathology. For the rest, if you provide the missing quality to your muscles—the pain goes away.

Keep in mind too that **function precedes form,** which means that before your body **looks** as if it were in trouble, it **acts** as though it were. A failure in any one of the first six tests means trouble brewing, trouble that must be fixed before you get on with the fun.

MINIMUM MUSCULAR FITNESS TEST

- *Start your program with this test.*
- *Retest every six weeks with special attention to test **2** and test **6**.*
- *If you fail in any area, do the exercises listed with the test.*
- *Failure to pass test 6 means that, besides being inflexible, you do not have sufficient physical activity to balance your emotional tension.* Height and build have nothing to do with it. *However there are mechanical faults that do.*
- *The Kraus-Weber test is a medically valid test for the* **minimum** *muscular fitness of your key posture muscles.*

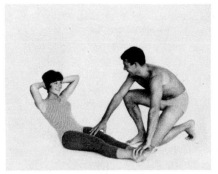

TEST 1. A+ (Abdominals plus help of psoas or hip flexors) Lie supine, legs held down, hands clasped behind neck. ROLL UP TO SITTING POSITION **ONCE.**

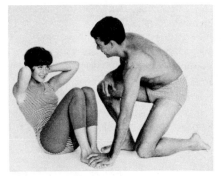

TEST 2. A— (Abdominals minus help of psoa or hip flexors) This is a truer abdominal tes Start supine with hands behind neck, **knee** **bent,** feet held down. ROLL TO SITTING POS TION **ONCE.**

If you failed either of these two tests your abdominals are weak. Do exercises 1, **2,** 3, 4, 5, 6, 7, 8.

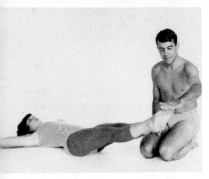

TEST 3. P (Psoas or hip flexors) Lie supine hands behind neck. RAISE BOTH LEGS ten inches from floor and hold for ten seconds. Count seconds by adding a three-syllable word to the number of the second, as, "one-chim-pan-zee, two-chim-pan-zees," etc. Try not to let your back arch unduly.

If you failed to hold the elevated position for 10 full seconds do exercise **17**.

TEST 4. UB (Upper Back) Lie prone over pillow, hands clasped behind neck, legs held down. RAISE UPPER BODY just off floor and hold for ten seconds. If you failed to hold your upper body up for ten seconds, do exercises **13** and **14**.

TEST 5. LB (Lower back) Lie prone over pillow, head resting on arms, upper body held down. RAISE BOTH LEGS from floor and hold for ten seconds. If you failed to maintain the lift, do exercises **13** and **15**.

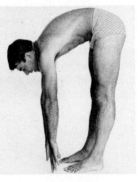

TEST 6. FLEX (Flexibility of back and hamstrings) With feet together, and knees straight, lean **over** and see how close you can bring fingertips to **floor**. NO BOUNCING OR KNEE BENDING. Measure **failure** in inches between fingertips and floor. If you could not touch the floor and hold the touch for three seconds, do exercises 67, 68, 69, 70. Do **74** several times daily.

OPTIMUM TEST

The MINIMUM test is exactly that. It's a start. It tells you in what ways you are good and exactly how good you are. For instance, it is encouraging to know that although you are inflexible, your back is strong, or perhaps vice versa—as long as you're never quite satisfied. You will want to chart your improvement; you will soon be involved with more than minimums.

Americans lack strength in hands, arms and shoulder girdle. Men in particular lack flexibility, as do at least 40% of youngsters age 16. Women lack strength, and almost everyone lacks high-level endurance. If you wonder why, just compare their daily sedentary activities with the active ones and you have the answer.

Now nobody is going to suggest giving up the car, the TV or the washing machine just so that you will become more "fit." We've come a long way since the days when the way we lived kept us in shape and no one wants to go back down **that** trail. On the other hand, if we don't do something about it, Americans will become more tired than they are already, and fatigue is one of the most common complaints people take to their doctors.

We will grow fatter. About 15% of our school children are obese; you can imagine what their parents look like.

Heart attack will become even more deadly than it is today. And the pursuit of happiness will grow obsolete as fewer and fewer are fit enough to go after it.

It is said that the average person uses less than one fifth of his brain capacity. It is undoubtedly true that he is just as remiss in the demands he puts upon his body. What does it all mean?

Never in his life does the average man or woman ask or get from the human body even a fraction of its potential. But any adult **at any age** who builds a body with anything like its true capability, may well find himself superior not only to those in his own age bracket, but superior physically to those far younger. If you want to badly enough, you can reach the age of retirement with the body of a very young person, a body that can take you anywhere, a body that can bring life to you in its fullness just when you have garnered enough experience to really bring something to life. Today at age 40, 50 or 60 a person can get into very good shape in six weeks. It takes the average out-of-shape teenager about two years to accomplish the same thing. If **you have ever had a good body during your lifetime, a fine one is still within your reach** if you have the determination to rebuild it. There are no limits.

OPTIMUM TEST TIPS

- *Find out before you start your program where you are on your fitness ladder.*
- *To be excellent in one area (strong in your legs), yet poor in others (poor in arm strength or flexibility), is to be only half a structure. First go after the weakness, then add to your plus areas.*
- *Push-ups should not be modified for women and girls. Americans could be as strong in this area as the people of other nations. It is an out-dated opinion, not a fact, that girls and women can't do push-ups.*
- *Back and hamstring inflexibility (test 12) is due primarily to tension and incorrect coaching. Again, body build has nothing to do with failure to pass.*

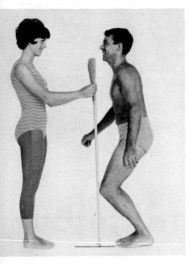

TEST 7. S. FLEX (Soleus and heel cord flexibility) Stand facing a wall, feet together about 2" from baseboard. Keep seat tucked under, heels flat on floor. Try to touch both knees to wall. If they touch easily, move feet back until you can just make it. Toes 4" from wall is very good. To improve, do exercises 30, **56**, 62a, 62b, 62e, 63a, 63c, 74.

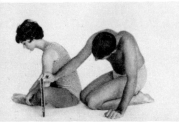

TEST 8. C. FLEX (Flexibility of those muscles leading down the legs from the crotch) Place soles of feet together and grasp ankles. Press down **evenly** on both knees with your elbows. Measure the distance from one knee to the floor. To improve, do exercises 43, 45, 67, 68, 69, **72**, 73.

TEST 9. PU (Push-ups) Lie prone, legs together, toes curled under, hands on floor near shoulder. Push up slowly, taking a full three seconds to reach full arm stretch. Descend as slowly, and when at rest on floor, swing hands around to touch each other above your back. This is one complete push-up. Repeat as often as you can, keeping body absolutely rigid. To improve, do exercises 19, **28**, 29, 30.

TEST 10. B. FLEX (Back flexibility) Place soles of feet together and pull your head down as close to feet as possible. Measure from forehead to floor. To improve, do exercises 67, 68, 69, **70, 71,** 74.

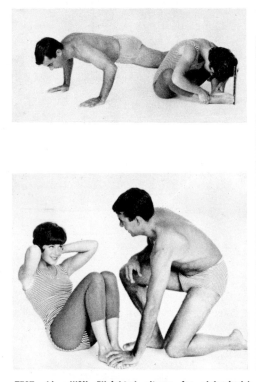

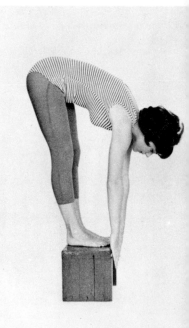

TEST 11. WSU (Weighted sit-ups for abdominals) On each succeeding sit-up, carry one more pound. If weight bags are not available carry an object heavy enough to limit you to ten sit-ups. If you use weight bags, score weight carried in last successful sit-up. If heavy object, score number of sit-ups. **To improve, do one-half your highest score twice daily. If using weight bags, carry one-half of your heaviest lift for ten sit-ups twice daily.**

TEST 12. B. & H. FLEX (Back and hamstring flexibility) Stand on a box and repeat TEST #6. Try to see how far you can reach down the side of the box without bending your knees. NO BOUNCING. Hold final reach for three seconds and record in plus inches. To improve, do exercises 67, 68, **69,** 71, 72, 73, 74.

16

MEASUREMENTS

While you are well aware that you must weigh yourself regularly (*see* OBESITY, *page* **153**), if you are to chart weight loss or gain correctly you can only plot the true picture by also **measuring** it. Muscle, while far more attractive than pudgy fat, actually weighs more than fat. So even if you exercise regularly and watch your diet carefully, your weight loss may not be impressive and you may get discouraged if you don't know what's happening.

Let's say that like most of us you don't exercise as much as you used to and you do eat more than you used to, yet the scale doesn't show an alarming weight gain. You may think you are one of the lucky ones who can get away with it. Then one day you get a good look at yourself in the mirror without your clothes on and you suddenly see what's wrong: You weigh the same but it's all run down into your protruding abdomen and thickened thighs. **You can never get away with it. These are the hard cold facts.**

1) If you exercise **and** diet correctly you will grow stronger and fat will disappear, leaving smooth, attractive muscle where it once bulged.

2) If you exercise but go on eating as before—or eating more—you will grow stronger but not necessarily slimmer.

3) If you don't want to lose weight but do want a better physique or a shapelier "more-of-you" body, as in the case of the girl who needs hips or bust (*see* CHEST & BUSTLINE *page* xx) or the man who wants a broader chest and heavier biceps, exercise doesn't take away muscle. It does take away fat. Where there isn't enough "you," you can build it.

4) If you want to lose weight but don't want to exercise, you are in for a disappointment. Take a look at those who have tried it. The weight came off all right, but the loose skin sags and droops. Haggard faces, neither filled in with fat nor good muscle tone, look old. Friends tell such people they looked better before they dieted (which may be true), so they give up trying.

5) If you want a new, better looking, more vital body, you will have to exercise **and** diet properly. To know exactly what is happening and where, you must measure. Keep track of all changes every six weeks. If you want it off of hips and it's coming off of waist and abdominals at too fast a rate, do more hip exercises. Be assured that there are specific exercises for particular areas of the body just as there are specific medicines for particular diseases. All the knee bends in the world won't make you more flexible, for example, any more than aspirin will help your hay fever. Decide what you want to change, then check in the TABLE OF CONTENTS for the exercise that will do the job.

MEASUREMENT TIPS

- *Know the shape of your shape as well as its weight and strengths.*
- *Measure every six weeks.*
- *Wear the same clothes (or preferably none) for each measuring.*
- *Menstrual periods will affect measurements (fluid retention).*
- *Muscle weighs more than fat, but is more attractive.*
- *Exercise will not give women and girls bulky muscles. Muscle gives girls curves.*
- *Addition of muscle via specific exercise can improve the bust line.*
- *Keep track of your addition and subtraction of inches, as well as pounds, it will be encouraging.*
- *It is quite true that a thin, weak, unattractive male body can be built into a very strong and attractive one in a fairly short time. Check improvement with the tape as the optimum test.*

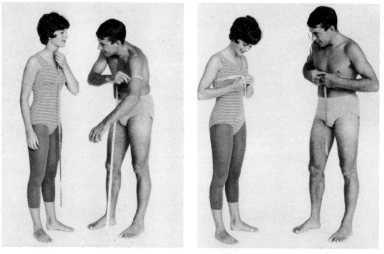

| NECK | ARMS | BUST | MID-RIFF |

NECK Measure the neck midway between shoulders and ears.
ARMS Relax arm when checking for flab; Measure 3″ from armpit. If checking for muscle, tighten fist and whole arm. Measure at greatest bulge.
BUST AND CHEST Inhale, then exhale half the air. Measure across nipples. Be sure tape is held level. If measuring for flab, stay relaxed. If measuring for muscle growth, press both fists together and tighten back and chest muscles.
MID-RIFF Move the tape down under the pectoral muscles or breasts and measure with lungs half empty.
ABDOMINALS Measure the bulge just below the navel.

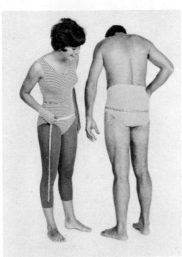
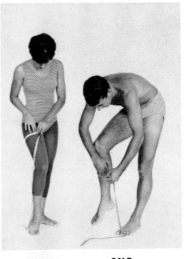

HIPS ONE   **HIPS TWO**   **THIGHS**   **CALF**

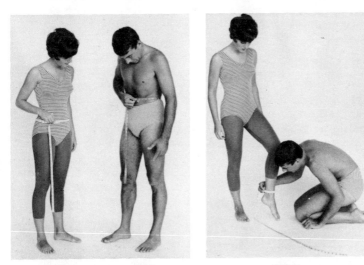

ABDOMINALS   **WAIST**   **ANKLE**

WAIST Don't pull in or tighten. You want to know the worst.
HIPS ONE (Mostly a woman's problem), measure at the side bulges and above the hips proper. Keep tape level.
HIPS TWO Measure the hips at their largest curve.
THIGHS When measuring for flab, unweight the leg and measure about 3″ from crotch. For muscle, straighten leg and tighten all down the leg. Measure at greatest bulge.
CALF For flab, unweight the leg and measure at largest curve. For muscle, stand on toe and tighten calf as you measure.
ANKLE Unweight leg and measure just above bony protuberance on inside of ankle.

19

YOUR HEART

Heart attacks kill the majority of men in America and they are striking younger and younger men. It is not unusual to lose a friend of 40 or 45. The fact that he was never sick a day in his life has no bearing on the case at all. He had been losing ground to that heart attack day by day for years.

Autopsies done on front-line soldiers killed in Korea (average age, 21) showed the majority had gross evidence of arteriosclerosis. In other words their arteries were already collecting deposits which would block one or another or many arteries. This means the blocked arteries could no longer carry blood to their areas of responsibility and those areas would, in effect, "die." While this might not be fatal, it would be painful and frightening and very damaging. If those arteries should be in the heart it could lead to a "coronary."

Most people are aware of "coronaries" but they often overlook the fact that the same process is going on in other parts of the body, including the brain. It's one thing to collapse like a light turned off at midnight, quite another to bumble along for years with parts of the brain permanently out of business.

It is known that diet (*see page* **154**) plays a tremendous part in the collection of substances that block arteries. Hundreds of studies have been made under controlled conditions, but probably the most dramatic was unplanned. During the war when eggs, milk, cream, butter and meat were hard to get, the number of deaths from "heart attacks" fell way off. After the war with the return to "normal" high-fat diets, coronaries zoomed. Read up on this dangerous situation if you are in charge of your family's food habits—or if you are a man who loves life. However, diet isn't all.

If you exercise regularly you can control obesity, a prime factor in heart disease and many other diseases as well. Exercise burns up the fat that would otherwise be stored to your detriment (and exercise affects the controversial cholesterol level).

Studies show that sedentary workers have twice as many heart attacks as active workers, and in the first attack, twice as many die. If you are an "active worker" you have built-in protection, just as women are protected by their sex hormones until menopause. Chances are you are not an active worker but there is nothing to prevent you from becoming good and active anyway by a simple regular program of exercise. To be sure it's **your** heart, but there are others involved. The average American woman lives eight years longer than her husband, and it can be very lonely. If you are a wife or a mother you can do more than anyone else to protect the men in your life. Feed them right. See to it that they exercise often, that their waistlines stay trim. Concern for their health should be oriented to **prevention** rather than repair. The lives you save may be the ones you love.

YOUR HEART—TIPS

- The heart is a muscle *and if it is healthy (as most are in the beginning) you can't exhaust it. Long, long before your heart would run out of steam your body's other muscles would collapse and leave you in a heap.* It is the unexercised heart *that is in danger, not the exercised or even over-exercised heart. Like all other muscles it benefits from use and deteriorates if it is not used often and completely.*
- Heart disease is on the increase *but not from overwork. It is caused by the wrong diet and by inactivity. When a man keels over from snow shoveling it isn't the shoveling that did the job, it was the years of inactivity and the wrong food.*
- You don't prevent an attack by resting and avoiding activity, *you prevent it with proper diet reversing the process that causes blocking in the arteries and by a steadily (but slowly) increasing program of activity.*

HEART CHECK

Test materials: box, pencil and notebook (in which you have already entered your muscular fitness test results, your measurements and your weight). Label a page with five columns.

Date

At rest	Standing	Action	After 1 minute	After 5 minutes

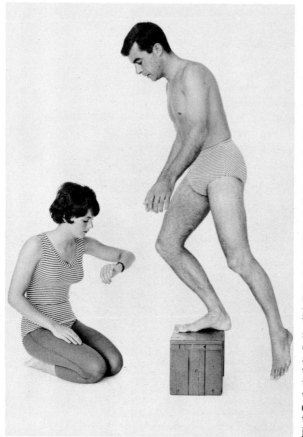

Lie flat for 10 minutes, then take your pulse; enter it under "AT REST." Stand up and take your pulse again; enter under "STANDING." Next find out what your heart does when it is put under a little pressure. In the course of one minute you should be able to step up onto a box with first one foot and then the other . . . and then step down the same way, 30 times (If you are in very poor shape settle for 15 times in half a minute). You are to take 2 full seconds for each up-down action, which consists of four separate steps. Step up on the right foot on the count of "one." On "two" step back down with the right foot. Do 30; immediately take your pulse. Enter under "ACTION." Rest for a minute and take it again. Enter the result under "AFTER 1 MINUTE." Rest for 5 more minutes and enter under "AFTER 5 MINUTES." Give yourself this test every 6 weeks. You will find that you return to the starting pulse rate faster as exercise improves your heart action and recovery rate. Don't take the test when you are under the weather even with a mild cold. Results will be inconclusive. To improve do the endurance exercises 96 through 103, particularly rope jumping.

ABDOMINALS

This area takes up a good part of you and is responsible for a great part of your well being. If your abdominals are weak and flaccid it is almost certain that the rest of you (both inside and out) is flaccid and weak as well. How can you tell? *When abdominals are weak, they protrude,* and when fat is present they protrude even further. Nothing you can wear will hide the fact that there is not only too much of you, but that it is mushy besides.

If you decide that diet is the only answer and you go ahead and diet stringently, you will lose weight and some of it is bound to come off the abdominals. Since you are doing nothing to improve the muscle tone and thus take up the slack as the fat disappears, you will be left literally holding the bag. There will be a great empty sack hanging down like a double-fold apron.

When the abdominals are weak the body is thrown out of line and undue pressure is put on muscles which are not equipped to handle the problem. The result is often back pain; 80% of all our *backaches* are caused by muscle deficiency, and weak abdominals are more often than not the troublemaker.

Allover fatigue is another by-product of weak abdominals: when they can't do their share in supporting the body and its contents, overworked muscles responsible for other jobs simply cannot cope with the extra burden, and fatigue is inevitable.

Weak abdominals indicate that the trunk is not being worked enough, and what they show on the outside other conditions prove on the inside. *Constipation* is one such indication. Even proper diet cannot do the job, and often people resort to medicines that become habit-forming. A by-product of constipation is painful *hemorrhoids*.

Cramps are another indication that the abdominal area has been allowed to become sluggish and swampy, lacking in good circulation and muscle tone. They are almost always unnecessary and usually can be prevented with the same exercises as those that improve the appearance of the abdomen.

Pregnancy is a severe test for abdominals. If tone is good and the muscles strong and elastic a woman rarely looks nine months pregnant until the end of nine months, and rarely even then. When tone is poor and the muscles weak the mother's appearance and posture are soon grotesque and almost invariably a backache becomes her constant companion. If she does get back her trim figure it's only after weeks and even months. After a second and a third pregnancy, her figure is only a memory. (Good abdominals are a great help during delivery.)

Incontinence (the inability to control the bladder) need not be drastic and total to cause a great deal of distress. Often after the birth of several children, women find the muscles of the pelvic area weakened. The simple act of running becomes not so simple and they are afraid to move suddenly or take part in anything involving jumping, such as an exercise or dance class, lest they "lose control." The abdominals play a part even here since their reconditioning helps to recondition other muscles, the ones which could do away with this embarrassing condition.

It may seem strange to connect *love-making* with abdominal muscles and yet it is impossible to leave them out of the picture. While there is no question that the ability to make love depends on other factors like sensitivity—and just being in love—still there is a physical side, and only the foolish or the ignorant ignore it. Strong resilient abdominal and back muscles improve love-making, and lack of either takes much pleasure away.

The *potbelly* seen today on even very young people, is usually the first sign of deterioration. The seldom exercised abdominals cannot wall in the contents of the abdomen. While women and girls may hide this condition for a little while with girdles (and men are beginning to use the same crutch) the weakness still exists. Instead of developing a strong elastic girdle of muscle which will keep the abdominals flat, strong and attractive . . . the girdle wearer pokes the pelvis into rubbery confines. Since this further limits the use of the muscles, the potbelly becomes even more pronounced and fat begins to gather. This means a larger "pot" and an ever larger girdle— or the feeling of suffocation.

Men do something even more disastrous. Since the disappearance of suspenders, many men hold up their trousers up by poking their abdominals out. That isn't their intention of course, but since the abdominals are flaccid, the "pot" is pronounced. Belt measurement gradually expands. Tightening the abdominals and pulling in hard would leave far too little pressure against the belt to support the trousers at the waist. Solution: low-rise trousers that permit the trousers' belt to be supported by the pelvic bone at either side— and exercise.

A potbelly means weak abdominal muscles. Weak abdominal muscles mean your body must be out of line. Being out of line inevitably leads to fatigue, and almost surely a backache. Correcting this problem will not only improve your appearance, it will help you keep your back in shape. If yours is already complaining, start to fix it by fixing your abdominals.

ABDOMINAL EXERCISE TIPS

- *Start with the test for minimum muscular fitness (on page 12) then add test 11 (on page 16).*
- *For weak abdominals do exercises 1, 2, 3, 4, 5, 6, 7, 8, 9, 10, 11.*
- *For fatigue do exercises 1, 2, 5, 6, 113, 114, 115.*
- *For constipation do exercises 1, 3, 4, 5, 6, 7, 8, 19, 33, 37.*
- *For hemorrhoids do exercises 1, 5, 6, 7, 8.*
- *For cramps do exercises 1, 2, 4, 5, 6, 7, 8, 17, 18, 19, 109.*
- *With pregnancy do exercises 104 through 112.*
- *For better love-making do exercises 1, 4, 5, 6, 7, 8, 17, 32, 38, 71, 72.*
- *For incontinence do exercises 1, 2, 5, 6, 7, 8.*
- *For pot belly do exercises 1, 2, 6, 7, 8, 17, 31, 33, 35.*

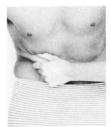

If there's more than half an inch, he's **fat!**

ABDOMINAL EXERCISES

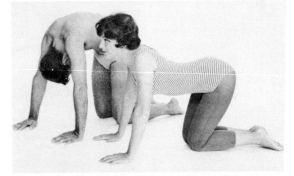

1 CAT AND OLD HORSE Start on hands and knees. Let your abdominals sag. Look at them, then without moving anything but your abdominals, tighten and pull them in hard. When they are as tight as you can manage, arch your back like an angry cat and tighten any inside muscles you can find. Hold for three slow counts, then bring your head up, allowing your back to sag like a tired old horse. Start with four of these, work up to eight.

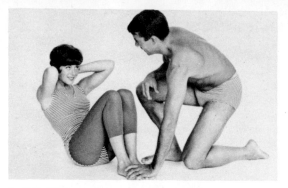

2 ROLL-DOWNS   Knees bent, hands behind neck, feet held down. Roll **slowly** down to lie on floor.

   If too difficult, start at top of ROLL-DOWN with arms stretched in front of you. Get up any way you can and repeat for ten. When that becomes easy, ROLL DOWN with hands across chest and fling arms forward to sit up. Later ROLL DOWN with hands behind neck and come up the same way. Do ten twice daily and check your progress with **Test 11.**

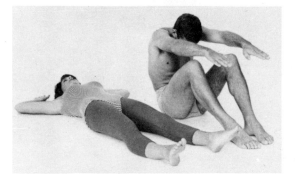

3 ROLL-OUTS Sit with legs spread, back round, chin on chest. ROLL OUT to spread position. Do four. Next try same with arms **stretched** forward, knees bent. If difficult, brace your feet under a heavy chair. Do four.

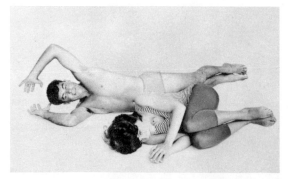

4 CURLS Can be done in bed before you get up. Lie on one side, knees pulled way up. Extend legs straight down and arms up. Stretch as far as you can and roll to other side. Curl tight and repeat. Do eight.

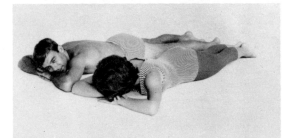

5 PELVIC TILT PRONE Lie prone and relaxed. First tighten your seat muscles (gluteals), pinch them together and hold. Next add the abdominal muscles. Hold the gluteals and abdominals "set" (try also to add the anal sphincter, the muscle that controls exacuation) for five slow counts. Relax and repeat four times.

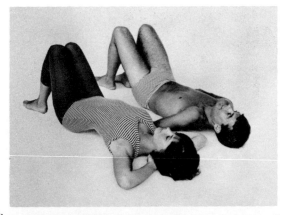

6 PELVIC TILT SUPINE Lie supine with knees bent, arms at rest. Arch back slightly and then with all your strength press spine flat on floor, which will have the effect of tilting your pelvis slightly forward. Tighten the anal sphincter and the internal sphincter which controls the bladder. Hold everything for count of five. Relax and repeat four times.

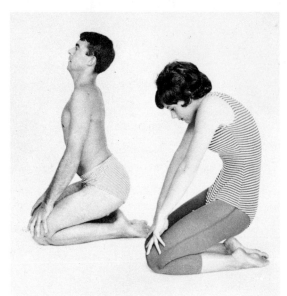

7 PELVIC TILT KNEELING Kneel with insteps flat on floor. (If impossible, thrust towel under ankles.) Start by arching back sharply, head up, chest well out. Now, without raising the level of your head, round back, drop head and tilt pelvis way under. Do four.

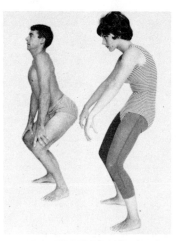

8 PELVIC TILT STANDING Stand with feet apart, knees bent. Arch back, raise head and thrust chest out. Next, round back, drop head and thrust pelvis forward and under. Don't straighten knees. Do eight.

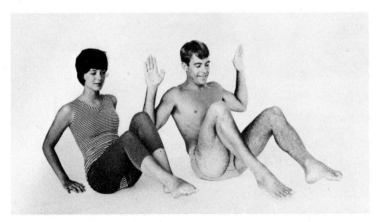

9 FOOT TAP Put on a fast record for this one. Start by resting weight back on your hands. Lift both feet simultaneously to tap to the rhythm. After sixteen such taps do the same, but tapping from side to side. These two actions make a series. Do four series.

When you are strong enough, lift hands from floor and do your tapping free of support.

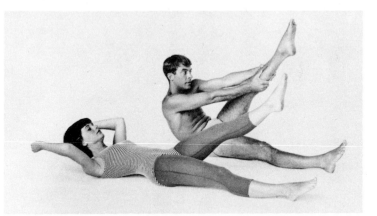

10 THE FLAGPOLE Lie supine with arms stretched overhead and raise one leg, **knee straight.** Swing arms forward as you sit up and grasp your leg wherever you can. Walk your hands up toward your ankle and then, leaving the leg suspended, lie back down. Do four with each leg for a series. Do three series. As soon as you can, give up the intermediate hand walking steps and try to swing up to catch the ankle with each sit up.

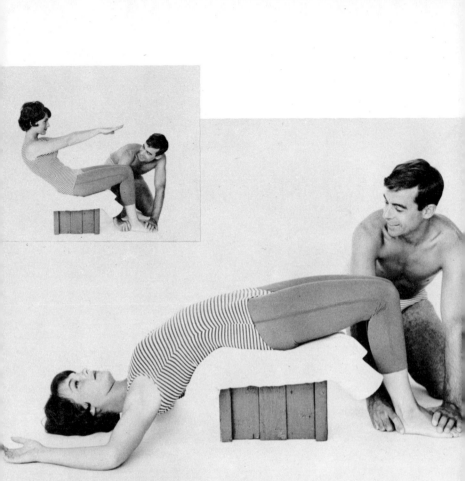

11 SIT-UPS FROM ARCH-DOWN This is an advanced exercise and should be treated with respect. Don't even consider it until you can do thirty bent-knee sit-ups **(Test 2).**

Place a pillow on a box. Higher the box, tougher the exercise. Sit on the box so that edge is a little below your waist as you lie back. Your feet should be anchored by somebody or something (a heavy chair will do). Extend arms forward to rest on thighs, drop your head and round your back. Roll **slowly** backward until head and shoulders come to rest on floor. (If box is high enough you may just hang arched and suspended.) Swing arms forward and roll up to sitting position. Start with two or three and work up to six, BUT TAKE YOUR TIME. To make this harder without increasing repetitions, hold weights (page 122) in hands. To make it still more difficult, don't swing the weights forward, but hold them behind neck.

BACKS

There is nothing like a backache to put you out of business, yet 80% of them could be and should be avoided. If you are not plagued already, are you a candidate for a backache? Ask yourself: Are you in a sedentary occupation? Do you try to make up for inactivity on weekends? Were you ever a competing athlete? Are you under any kind of stress? Are you a tense, driving sort of person? Did you ever have a bad fall? Are you overweight? Do you have a posture problem? Do you stand all day on the job? Sit all day? Do you have a garden? Children? Do you drive a car long distances? Do you sleep in a soft bed? Have troubles begun to pile up?

If you had to answer yes to even a few of those questions your chances for a bout with acute backache are good. Backache rarely occurs all by itself, unless you just fell down a flight of stairs. There is almost never a backache that just "appears" unless there is considerable *stress* beforehand.

Inflexibility is the cause of many backaches. If you fail test #6 or have difficulty with #7 and #10, you are inflexible. That means your muscles are not fully stretched to give you full range of motion. When these inflexible muscles pull you out of line as they do in *swayback, roundback, flatback* or *curvature*, they not only bring on pain, but fatigue as well. If any of these conditions are coupled with weak abdominals, you are in for it.

Weakness contributes its share to the misery of backache. When muscles cannot do the work for which they were designed others must step in and help; muscles that were not meant to serve in a prolonged emergency soon tire, leaving you unprotected against any sudden crisis.

While there are many reasons for backache, only 20% come under the heading of pathology. The other 80% are caused by muscle deficiency *plus stress*. When a doctor says you haven't a "ruptured disc" and you haven't "arthritis of the spine" and it isn't "rheumatism" and your back isn't "out," he does not mean to imply that it's all in your head. All he means is there's nothing on the X-ray and he can't find anything he can recognize that could cause such pain. Yet you know you have a backache.

Usually this is what has happened. A muscle, quite often in the gluteal (seat) region or in the muscles surrounding the 4th and 5th lumbar vertebrae (lower back), goes into spasm—it forms into a tight little knot. This is painful and leads to further spasm, which in turn leads to more pain. When the pain becomes acute enough, neighboring muscles add spasms of their own to the clamor, and sometimes a muscle as far removed from the seat of the problem as the upper back and even in the lower leg may be heard from. Backs with their intricate system of nerves are hard to peg. The spasm-pain-spasm cycle begins and it won't stop until the cycle is interrupted by medication, injection, skin surface coolant or something with heat, preferably wet.

But what, you wonder, set off the initial spasm in the first place? That's where old injuries come in. They leave tight spots in the muscle and it seems that as long as you leave them alone, they leave you alone *unless you are under stress.* That stress could be sitting too long at a work table, piano, desk or the wheel of a car. It could be the tension of a job or unhappiness, or the carrying of too much weight. It could even be the unaccustomed strain of snow shoveling or gardening when you aren't in shape for it, and without warning that old injury begins to tighten up. At first it isn't noticeable, or perhaps later there may be some discomfort. Then one morning you lean over to pick up the paper and zing! Your back is "out." The truth is it isn't really "out" and it doesn't go back in. It's in spasm and that's bad enough. All you can do about it at the moment is get to your doctor, get some medication and do what he says until the acute phase is over. After that you had better get to work on preventing another such unpleasant occasion. It can almost always be done.

Occupations have a lot to do with the way a back behaves and so does the sport of your choice. For instance if your back is acting up and the doctor says it's muscle deficiency, don't rush right out and play three sets of tennis to get it into shape. Tennis, like volley ball, handball, even golf, is a "spike" sport with unpredictable starts and stops (a slice is certainly unpredictable!). You have to tighten many muscles including that sensitive one . . . and that's what you don't want to do. Certain exercises are corrective, others, like "jumping jacks" and running in place, are not. (See *Occupational Hazards* on page **146**.)

Muscle fatigue leading to backache can be brought on by inactivity as often as by overactivity. When you must hold muscles in one position too long they do not get the rest and relaxation provided by being relieved of their tension while others go into action. A simple way of avoiding muscle fatigue is to work by the clock rather than the job. Ten minutes of weeding, ten of carting, ten spent on the stone fence, ten in following the lawn mower, and then back to the weeding. I call it "smorgasbord working," and it looks both haphazard and disorganized. But the work will get done, and you will avoid "Monday Misery." The same applies to housework; even the dentist can schedule his hours so that the difficult tense work is spelled by other tasks.

Habits can cause a backache (and almost any other ache as well). Do you sit on one foot? Do you sit curved to one side in the car? Is your desk chair wrong for you and do you make a habit of compensating for it? Do you always carry books or a briefcase in the same hand? Does a handicap such as deafness pull your head and shoulders one way as you strain to hear? Check out your habits and see if they are factors in recurring backache.

Pregnancy can cause backache if back muscles are not flexible and abdominals are not strong. If you find yourself at this moment in the middle of such an event, that is no excuse. Begin at once with the exercises on pages **134–137**.

There are mechanical reasons for backache too. Many of us are born with one side smaller than the other. This may show up in the structure of the face, by a shoulder which droops, one breast which is slightly smaller or a downward tilt to one side of the waist. 77% of us have one leg that is shorter than the other, some as little as ¼ of an inch. While this small discrepancy is considered by doctors to be "clinically unimportant" it can assume considerable importance if it couples with long hours of standing on cement floors. Should the lower back be under stress from injury or any form of prolonged stress, ¼ of an inch may be just enough to throw the back into the spasm-pain-spasm cycle.

Should the unequal torso (which means that the pelvis is also unequal and the "sitting bones" cannot strike the chair evenly) be subjected to the occupational stress of long hours in a sitting position, it too can contribute to backache. Since the upper back and neck are affected by any imbalance in either the legs or the torso, stiff necks, shoulders, and arms may result . . . as well as headaches, vaguely complaining molars and even dizzyness.

As an aid to correct the smaller side, sit with a magazine (the *Reader's Digest* is usually the right size and unobtrusive) under the buttocks on the small side. To lengthen a "clinically unimportant" but troublesome short leg, put a ¼ inch pad in the heel of the shoe. If you need more, add leather to the bottom of the heel. For boots and sandals, have the whole sole built up.

We always have some stress with us, but occasionally it gets out of hand. The quick crisis, no matter how difficult or painful, is far less dangerous to a back than a long, slow, grinding problem in which the sufferer must try to adjust over and over again to an all but unbearable situation. This is seen when a person is in the throes of a divorce (the divorce doesn't do the damage, the preceding months or years of stress are responsible), or when some family situation is untenable. If you are in some unhappy circumstance make sure you have enough physical outlet for the release of tension so it doesn't take itself out on your back.

Fibrositis is a by-product of stress and your entire back is fair game. It occurs when areas of muscle are constantly and unconsciously tightened under stress, rage, frustration, or just extended concentration. The shoulders, neck and thighs show it by thickened tissue, but the back *feels* it. (*See Fibrositis on pages* **104–107**).

At no time in life can anyone afford to ignore a bad back. Too many nerves go through there and too much of the rest of you depends on it. Check yours for flexibility (*Test #6*) and for weakness (*Tests #4 and #5*) and for fibrositis and for ache (you needn't look that one up), then start to put yours in order. In *any* case do the back series beginning on page **35**.

BACK EXERCISE TIPS

- *Most backaches are avoidable; 80% can be done away with through proper exercise.*
- *For backache* not *due to pathology, do exercises* **12a, 12b, 12c, 12d, 12e,** *plus* **74.**
- *For inflexibility, do exercises 12a, 12b, 12d, 16, 31, 33, 37, 67, 68, 69, 70,* **74.**
- *For upper back weakness, do exercises* **13a,** *13c, 13e, 13f, 14.*
- *For lower back weakness, do exercises* **13b,** *13d, 13e, 13f, 15, 37, 38, 39, 80.*
- *With pregnancy, do exercises on pages 134 thru 137.*
- *For fibrositis, see exercises 64a–e.*
- *For stress, see "warm-ups" on page 142.*
- *For poor posture, see Posture Section page 41.*
- *For backache connected with occupations, see* Occupational Hazards, page *146.*
- *For lower back pain, do exercises 12a, 12b, 12c, 12d, 12e, 16, 20, 21, 22, 23, 26, 27, 31, 33, 115.*
- *For fat back do exercises 13a, 13b, 13c, 13d, 13e, 13f, 14, 15, 19, 23, 27, 30, 31, 33, 34, 35, 37, 39.*

LIMBERING EXERCISE SERIES FOR BACKS

This series of exercises is designed to make back muscles limber and to strengthen abdominal muscles. These are the first steps after the doctor says, "Try exercise first." They prevent muscle spasm. Their gentle but persistant use will gradually untie the knots. If your backache was bad enough to send you to a doctor ask him first **when** you may try these exercises.

To **prevent** muscle spasm this series must be done often throughout the day **before** warning of pain informs you that a spasm is starting. Begin before you get out of bed. Schedule another series for noon, mid-afternoon, evening and night.

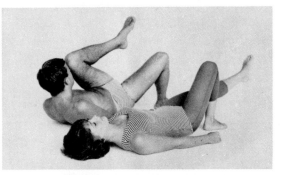

12a SINGLE KNEE KISS Lie supine, knees bent. Bring one knee as close to nose as possible, then extend leg and let your head fall back to rest position. Finish in bent-knee position. Alternate four each leg and roll over onto your other side.

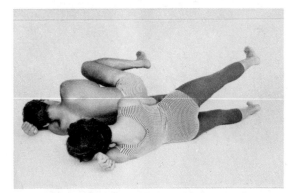

12b KNEE-TO-CHEST Draw top knee up as close to your chest as possible. Now extend leg to a position a few inches above the other leg . . . then lower to rest position and relax. Do four slowly, with plenty of rest between. Then roll face-down.

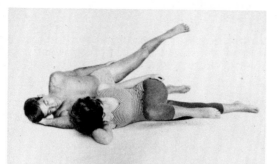

12c KNEE-TO-CHEST ON OTHER SIDE Repeat knee-to-chest-extend action you already did, this time with other leg. Do four times. Then roll into position from which you started.

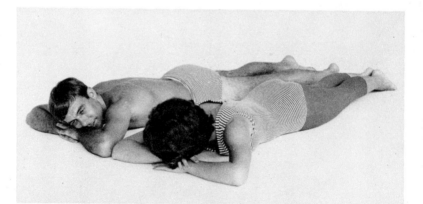

12d ABDOMINAL & GLUTEAL SET Tighten seat muscles (gluteals) and hold. Next, tighten abdominal muscles, pulling in hard. Hold gluteal and abdominal set for slow count of five, then relax for slow count of three. To further relax the seat, allow heels to fall outward, toes together. Do four.

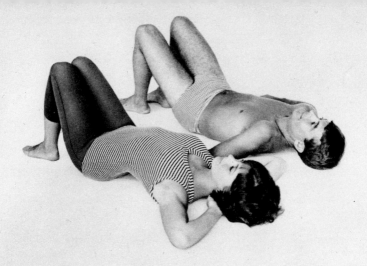

12e PELVIC TILT SUPINE
Arch your back a little first, then press spine down hard against floor. Hold for slow count of five, relax for three and repeat. Do four.

Do whole series twice but take your time. Keep in mind that there is rarely a backache without tension, and you are trying to relax yours.

EXERCISES FOR BACK STRENGTH

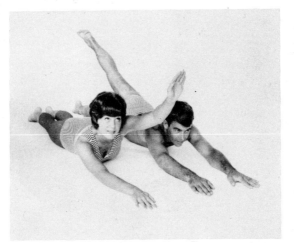

13a ARM RAISES Lie prone with arms and legs outstretched. Raise one arm **slowly** and then as **slowly** lower it. Do not roll chest from side to side; let all the action be in arm and shoulder. Alternate, four each side.

13b LEG RAISES Lie prone with straight legs, arms outstretched. Raise the one leg **slowly** and as **slowly** lower it. Alternate, four each side.

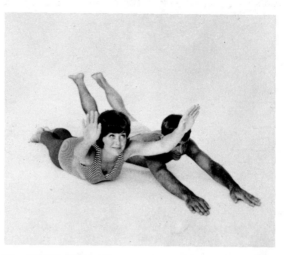

13c DOUBLE ARM RAISE Lie prone with arms and legs outstretched. Raise both arms as high as possible and hold for slow count of three. Lower. Do four.

13d DOUBLE LEG RAISE (If you notice heavy strain with this exercise, do it over a pillow as in tests #4 and #5). Lie prone, arms and legs outstretched. Raise both legs and hold for a slow count of three. Lower. Do four.

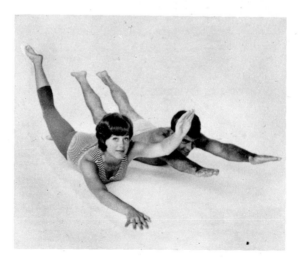

13e ALTERNATE ARM & LEG RAISE Lie prone, arms and legs outstretched. Raise **right** arm and **left** leg at same time. Lower and repeat with **left** arm and **right** leg. Do four of each.

13f DOUBLE ARM & LEG RAISES Lie prone, arms and legs outstretched. Raise **both** arms and **both** legs at same time. Lower. Do four.

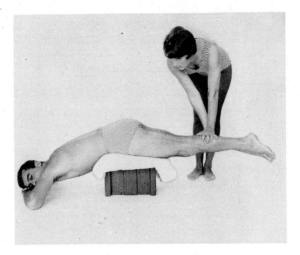

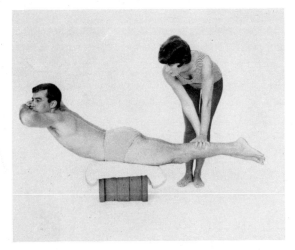

14 UPPER BACK LIFTS OVER SUPPORT Lie prone over a box (or the edge of a table or bed) with legs weighted. Rest head and arms on floor and RELAX. Raise head and upper body to a level a little higher than the hips. Hold for slow count of four and lower. Do four. To make this more difficult, extend arms. Still more difficult, carry weights in hands.

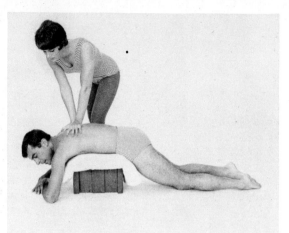

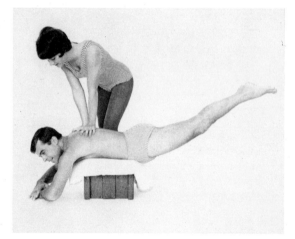

15 LOWER BACK LIFTS OVER SUPPORT (This can be done without help by leaning over a table and holding onto the other side). Lie prone over a box with upper body held down. Raise both legs to a level a little above the hips and hold for a slow count of four. Do four. To make this easier, lift one leg at a time. To make it harder, use weights.

POSTURE

The way you stand, sit, move and even rest, tells more about you than your signature—and it's harder to disguise. Your fears, hostilities, anxieties, weariness, despair and even your loneliness can be seen in your walk. Oddly enough, when you change these outward signs of inner tension you can often improve your ability to handle the tensions themselves.

Your posture habits began to form as soon as you began to sit up, to stand and to walk. Very often active children, pulling themselves up on chairs, tables and the bars of cribs and playpens develop **sway backs,** because from the start they develop the habit of standing with chest out, bottom out and tummy poked forward. If **you** have a sway back know that a habit probably started it and that Ex #16 can probably correct it.

The child who finds life a frightening experience or the child who is extremely shy often carries the signs through the rest of life in the shape of a **round back** or **stoop shoulders.** He begins by trying to pull back into himself; the shoulders round, stretching the upper back muscles until they are overstretched like worn-out rubber bands. The chest, pulled in constantly, shrinks and the chest muscles (pectorals) become short and tight. When parents and teachers say "stand up," he can't because of weakness in the back and constant pull in the front. This is exactly what is happening when the round-shouldered adult tries to "stand up" to relieve the pull and pressure and to get a full breath of air for a change.

The **sway back** stands with a sag inward at the waist. His seat pokes out behind and his abdominals balance this by poking out in front. There is meant to be some curve forward in the spine at that point, but not **that** much curve. As a consequence, the pelvis is tipped backward putting great strain on the muscles around the 4th and 5th lumbar vertebrae.

The opposite of **sway back** is the **flat back.** It is less well known and it is not quite as obvious, but it causes just as much backache, fatigue and is very hard to clothe. In the **flat back** the spine is too straight where the **sway back** is too curved. There is almost a straight line down the back from shoulder blades to tail bone. Neither skirts nor pants hang well and it interferes with both appearance and good function.

Curvatures, known as **scoliosis** (when the line of the spine departs from straight up and down and curves to one side or the other) or **kyphosis** (when the upper curve of the spine is exaggerated to make an extreme round back) cause no end of worry.

Some of these departures from the normal have known causes, as for example polio, in which one set of muscles may not recover their full strength and allow the unaffected muscles, which are much stronger, to pull the bones out of line. There are many cases of curvature in which no cause can be traced, yet the results are the same: the body is out of line. In such cases, and there are many, they usually begin to show up at the age of 11 or at the start of puberty. They usually "set" and go no further at 17.

Forward head is an unattractive posture fault that gives the body an awkward look, causes neck and shoulder pain, headaches and fatigue. In this case there is usually a round back to start it off. The back rounds, the chest muscles shrink (try those two actions) then the person tries to look straight ahead. (Try that too, and you will find that the only way to get your head up is to thrust it forward.) Held that way long enough it will stay that way.

For extreme curvatures it is important to see a doctor especially if you have pain or are in those years between 11 and 17. Sometimes the simple addition of a lift in one shoe like the one Dr. Travell designed for President Kennedy, is enough to relieve the imbalance that causes substitution, compensation—and pain. If the curvature has "set," however, you should try to do as many exercises as possible that use **both** arms. Swimming is ideal, so are gymnastics. Tennis would be bad if it pulls too much and causes pain. If it is extreme round back that bothers you, think what is doing it— tight pectorals; they must be stretched. If a forward head goes along with it, pectoral stretch is first: Lie on a narrow bench and do Exercise #92, letting the weights pull those chest muscles open. Just let the arms hang for a few seconds; rest and repeat. Add neck stretches: Just slide up on the bench until its edge, protected by a pillow, rests under your shoulder blades. Let your head hang back as you let your hands hang down. You should look like you were going into a swan dive. Do this often throughout the day . . . use the time when the commercials are blatting on TV. Just have your bench or footstool, or ottoman and your weights handy . . . and stretch.

The **protruding abdomen** seems to appear whenever the back is out of line. As you correct the back and shoulder problems and strengthen your abdominal muscles, it tends to disappear.

POSTURE TIPS

- *Sway back (lumbar lordosis) occurs when the pelvis is tipped (so that measurements of the angle of the forward pelvic tilt show figures lower than 160°). This posture fault puts extra strain on all the muscles in the lower back and leads to fatigue as well as back pain. Do exercises 5, 6, 16,* **17.** *(In doing 16 do not exaggerate the "Old Horse" exercise; be content to let the back remain in a level position.)*

- *Flat back is the opposite of sway back. (Measurements of the pelvic angle measuring higher than 170° indicate a flat back.) The penalty for this posture fault is the same as for the sway back: fatigue and a good chance of backache, plus a probable clothes fitting problem. Do exercises 7, 8, 11, 18, 19.*
- *Round back (also called "Round Shoulders") causes shortening of the chest muscles (pectorals) and over-stretching of the upper back muscles. This causes increased tension and limits lung action. Do exercises 13a, 13c, 13e, 13f, 19, 26, 27, 30.*
- *Curvatures should not be ignored in the hope that they will go away. See your doctor for special exercises designed to develop the weaker areas and for possible mechanical correction.*
- *Protruding abdomen . . . same as for sway back.*

POSTURE CORRECTION

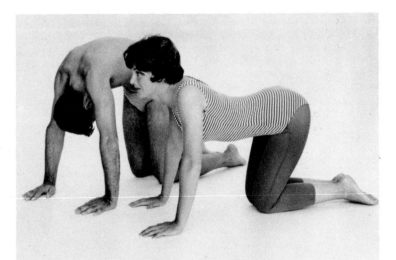

16 CAT AND OLD HORSE (This exercise is good for both SWAY BACK and FLAT BACK). Start on hands and knees. Keeping arms absolutely straight, press back up into angry cat position and drop head. Stretch your back as hard as you can. Hold position for slow count of four, then lower. If you have a sway back do not drop your back below the level position—no point in encouraging that sway. But if you have a flat back, do both the cat and the old horse. From arched angry cat position, allow back to fall into a sag. Repeat exercise four times. Alternate with exercise **17** and do four more.

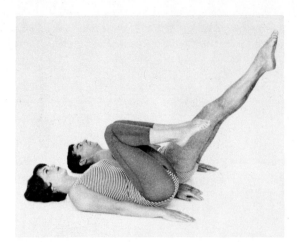

17 SPINE-DOWN STRETCH Lie supine, arms at sides, knees drawn up. Thrust legs straight overhead **keeping spine flat against the floor**. Legs should form a right angle to your body. Return to starting position and repeat, but on second extension, lower legs slightly as in the picture. **Be sure spine is flat on floor.** Keep returning to starting position and extending legs, each time a little lower, until you reach a point where you can no longer keep the spine flat. Then go back to the last successful spine-down stretch and do ten. Alternate with exercise **16** and then do ten more.

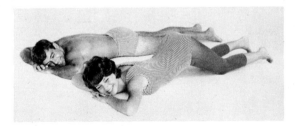

18 HIP LIFT Lie prone with chest tight to floor. Raise hips as high as possible, then lower. Do eight.

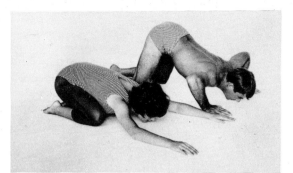

19 PEANUT PUSH Start on hands and knees, insteps flat on floor, seat just above heels, arms outstretched and chest as close to floor as possible. Open knees so that you can press your chest down still further. Start by pretending to push a peanut across the floor with your chin, sliding upper body slowly forward, **keeping your head down.** At full stretch, arch your back downward as you bring your head up. Finish by dropping head and pushing back through the ANGRY CAT position to the starting point. Start with four, work up to eight.

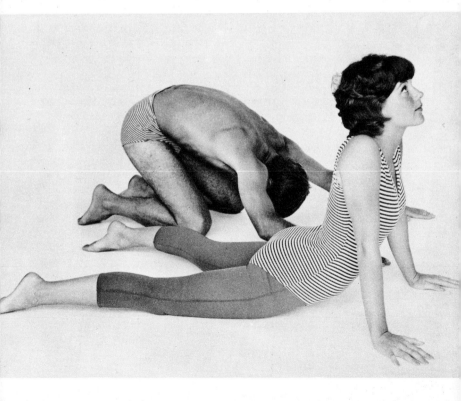

NECK

The muscles of the neck and those which spread upward into the head and downward over the shoulders and upper back are prime target areas for tension. Without realizing it many people tense these muscle areas when under any kind of stress. While the tightening may be both unconscious and imperceptible, it is still going on and the neck and shoulder muscles, just like the back muscles, will take only so much and then go into spasm. This produces the typical stiff neck (thought to be caused by a draught in the car when you were really too tense while driving).

All too often the neck is merely a way station from which further spasm travels up over the head to end as a pounding "tension headache" just above the eyes.

There are two cable-like muscles on either side of the neck that play an unsuspected part in many miseries. They have the name **sterno-mastoid** for the two points where they tie in. You can see them if you look in the mirror and turn your head from side to side. They start right back of the ears (mastoid process) and run down toward the center of the top of your chest (sternum). An injury to one or the other or even both of these, say in an accident that snaps your head, can go on and on long after other wounds heal. A little spasm **(trigger point)** hidden there can cause dizziness and a lack of balance. If the original accident included a head injury, imagination with the help of worried relatives can cause all sorts of havoc. Sometimes pain can be **referred** from the sterno-mastoid into the upper part of the chest and this gives the heart-conscious sufferer untold agonies.

Such important muscles . . . (after all they are involved with every move of your head) . . . have many ways of advertising their distress. They can make your molars ache in vague ways which mystify the dentist who can't find a thing wrong with them. Some people lose perfectly good teeth this way. They can even limit the size of the opening of your mouth. People with head or neck injuries often cannot open wide enough to insert **three** fingers curled into a fist. People without such injuries almost always can. Nobody realizes this, as when they open their mouths "wide" . . . they believe it **is** wide, no matter how small the opening. Try it yourself.

THE NECK TIPS

- *Most stiff necks are the result of tensing neck muscles unconsciously under stress. Do exercises **20, 21, 33.***
- *Once neck pain starts it is a sign that spasm has already begun in the muscle . . . try to* prevent *the spasm from starting by tying exercise **20** to habits you must follow throughout the day. Any habit will do—washing dishes or hands, putting a new sheet of paper into the typewriter, hanging up the receiver—anything, as long as it occurs at spaced intervals all day.*
- *If your neck is "tight" try to have someone do fibrositis massage on it every evening before you go to bed (exercises **64a,** 64b).*
- *Try not to hold your head still any longer than you must. Whenever possible do your work in smorgasbord fashion (see* Backs).
- *Don't wait until pain announces that spasm is already in action. Prevent the tightening by doing neck loosening exercises often throughout the day (pages **48–49**) and by using fibrositis in massage every night (pages **104–105**).*

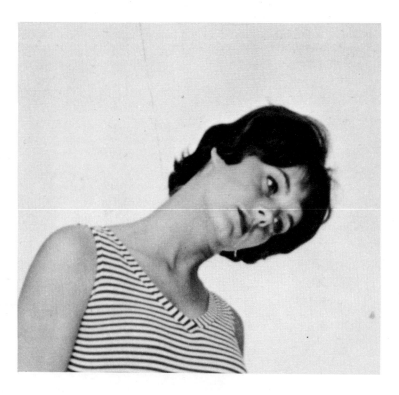

NECK EXERCISES

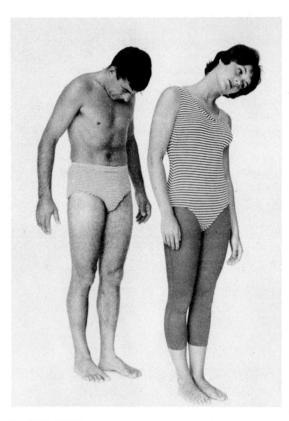

20 NECK ROLLS Drop head forward onto chest. Let weight
of head pull and stretch muscles at back of neck. **Just hang
limp.** After a few seconds you will notice a pulling sensation
first at the back of your neck, then down your spine almost
to your waist. Try consciously to "let go" at points where you
feel strain. Place hand on back of head and press head downward gently in little bounces to stretch the pulling muscles.

Then roll head to left side. There will be less strain when
your head is hanging a little in front of or in back of true
left. (If "true left" were at 9 o'clock, your head would feel
easier when you rotated it to 7 and 10 o'clock.) Roll it slowly
back and forth between 7 o'clock and 10 o'clock trying hard
to "let go" each time you pass the tight point at 9 o'clock.

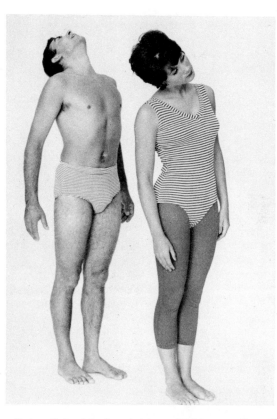

Next, roll head back and let mouth fall open. You will feel the pull at your throat and a bunched-up feeling at the back of your neck. Try hard to "let go" wherever there is pain. Let head hang back for about ten seconds, then roll it.

As head rounds the curve of true right there may be pain from tight areas and maybe even disturbing crunching sounds. No, your bones aren't coming apart. Keep rolling gently over this spot and eventually it will move smoothly without tension or complaint.

This is good exercise for double chin, but don't count on it to work alone. If chin and face are to be toned, all the rest of you will have to be toned as well.

SHOULDERS

Shoulders, like the neck and back, are targets for tension. You will find that whenever you are under considerable stress you tend to "bunch" your shoulders just as you would your fists if you expected a physical attack. A good "chewing out" on the job can cause it. So can heavy unrelieved concentrating on the job to be done. Check yourself after a long day behind the desk or the wheel of your car (especially if there was night driving on an expressway). Ever notice how, after a difficult day on the telephone, you can't seem to get your shoulders to "let go?"

Sometimes the first sign comes after the fact. The shoulder muscles have already started to spasm and you feel a warning sliver of white hot pain just back of the shoulder slope and about four inches to one side of the spine. From that moment on it can only get worse no matter what you do. The best thing would be to quit, go lie down, forget the job—but who ever can?

If repeated tension is borne too long the attacked tissue begins to thicken. You have probably seen this on older women, many times so thick it looks like a solid lump in the middle. This is called "Dowager's hump." It is **fibrositis** (*see pages* **104** *and* **105**), and to get rid of it the thickened tissue must be massaged with a very uncomfortable "pinching" action which in effect, "breaks the stuff up." That gives the exercise that must follow a chance to smooth out the affected areas and make them pliable again.

SHOULDER TIPS

- *Shoulders, like the neck and back, are tension targets.*
- *The best way to prevent tension from causing muscle spasm in the shoulders is to do exercises often throughout the day, exercises that will loosen and stretch muscles that are constantly being unconsciously drawn upward. Do exercises* **21,** *22 and 23 often during the day.*
- *Shoulder fibrositis is a thickening of the tissue when muscles are held tight too long and too often. To relieve this do exercises 21, 22,* **26.**
- *Round shoulders need chest stretch, do exercises* **26** *and* **27.**
- *For almost any sport using arms, shoulder flexibility is a must. Do exercises* **26** *and* **27.**
- *When shoulders have been injured and the doctor says "exercise" use* **24** *and* **25.**

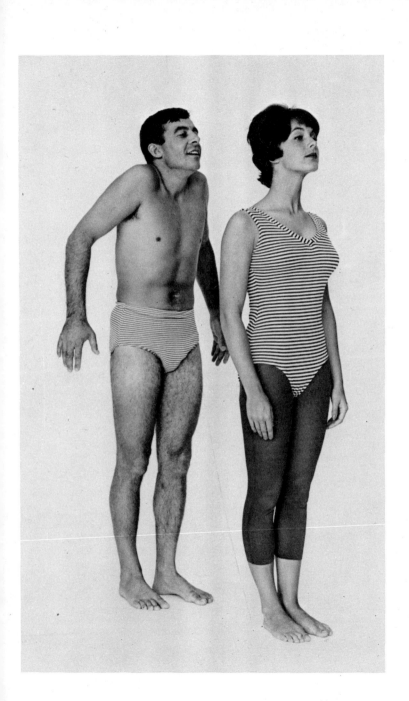

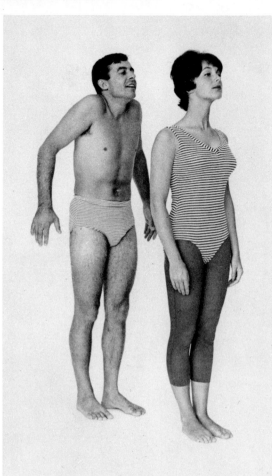

21 SHOULDER SHRUGS Pull shoulders up trying to "cover your ears." Pull hard and hold for five slow counts. Now allow shoulders to drop down to "make a long neck." Then push them even further down until you feel discomfort at back of neck and shoulders. Hold for five.

Now press shoulders forward to stretch all muscles across your upper back. You will feel this in your chest as the

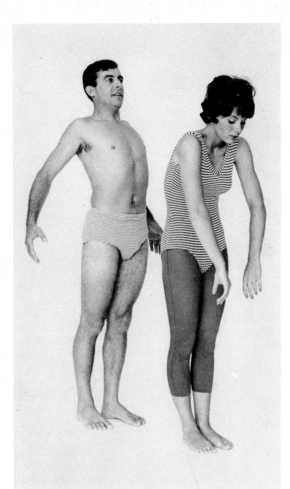

pectorals contract. Hold for five. Finally, thrust shoulders way back and lift both head and chest. Feel as though your shoulder blades are pressing against each other. Hold for five.

These four movements make one series. Do four series whenever you get a chance throughout the day. If there is only time for one such series at the change of tasks, take that time and make it pay off by working the muscles hard.

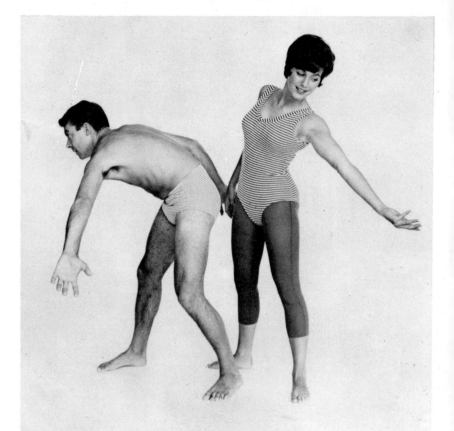

22 ARM AND SHOULDER ROTATIONS (If **fibrositis** is one of your problems do the massage pictured in **64b** and also apply the same principle to the backs of your arms **before** doing the exercise). Start with feet apart for balance. Twist right arm inward bringing not only the arm into play, but shoulder and whole upper body. You should feel the pull down as far as your waist. Next, turn arm all the way out, twisting your hand so that thumb points backward. Do four rotations with each arm, then do both arms at the same time to make up a series. Alternate with **exercise 36**. Both these exercises go well to a hot "Pop" beat.

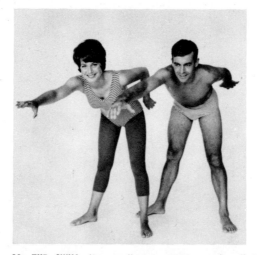

23 THE SWIM (An excellent warm-up exercise that should be done before almost any physical activity; it loosens upper body and increases blood flow to extremities.) Stand with feet wide apart. Use an alternating over-arm swim stroke reaching forward as far as possible. Do eight strokes, then turn upper body to right and do eight. Turn to left for eight more and finish with eight facing forward. Do two such series.

SHOULDER REPAIR EXERCISE

Any joint that is awkwardly or incorrectly used over a period of time or during extreme crisis will suffer. If your doctor says "exercise it" these will help.

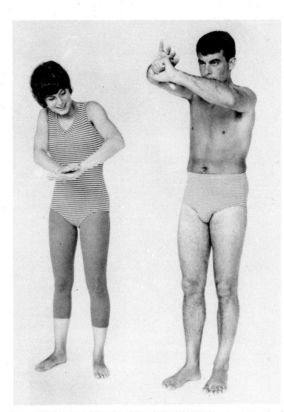

24 RESISTANCE LIFT FOR ARM AND SHOULDER Rest hand of complaining shoulder on back of "good" hand. Slowly and evenly to prevent discomfort that would cause shoulder to tense, raise "bad" arm as high as you can without gritting your teeth. Then from the top of lift **press downward** with "bad" hand. Pressure **down** with the "bad" hand will eventually give it more **upward** range. Repeat four or five times every few hours to get rid of stiffness.

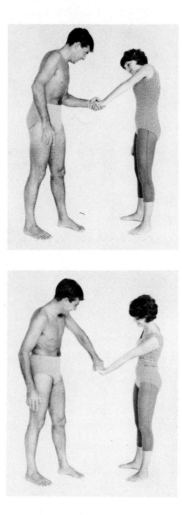

25 RESISTED ARM AND SHOULDER ROTATION (This will help so-called
"tennis elbow.") Take the other person's hand as if about to shake hands.
Rotate clasped hands inward and outward without resistance to set up a
pattern. Then on fourth rotation, person with the "good" hand sets up a
little resistance so that the other must work a little to keep the rotations going. Slowly increase pressure. Do ten or twelve with each session
and have a session every few hours.

Old injuries that cause stiffness and pain with weather changes
and enforced inactivity, such as desk work or driving, often respond to
rotations against resistance.

SHOULDER FLEXIBILITY EXERCISE (Also Round Back, Chest and Bustline)

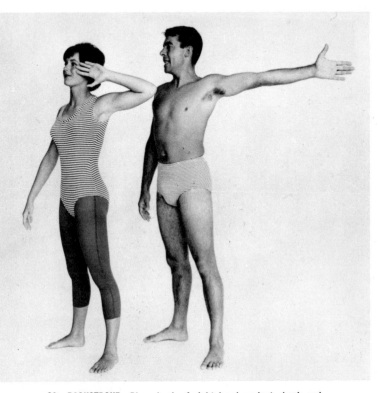

26 BACKSTROKE Place back of right hand against cheek and press elbow back as far as you can. You should feel a tightness in your shoulder blade. Keeping elbow back so that tight feeling does not diminish, straighten your arm so that the hand is reaching straight back. Be sure upper body faces straight forward and does not twist to right. When arm is at full stretch, bring it down to your side and repeat to the left. Alternate for eight. Then do both arms at the same time for eight. To make more difficult use weights (pages 122-128).

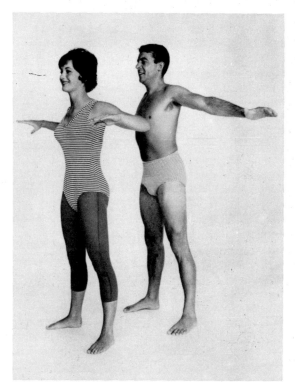

27 SNAP & STRETCH Raise bent arms to shoulder level and bring hands together in front so that fingers touch or overlap. With a sharp jerk, snap elbows back (you will feel your shoulder blades touch). Now bring hands together as before, then swing arms wide apart. Keep up a steady rhythm without a break. It should go SNAP-together-STRETCH-together-SNAP . . . The hands come together with each "together." Do four sets of eight. To make more difficult, carry weights.

CHEST AND BUST LINE

The chest of a man and the bust line of a woman have a great deal to do with the over-all appearance of both. For men, the size and shape of the chest has nothing to do with either vitality or virility but the well developed, muscular, wide chest bespeaks both, while the concave or narrow chest denies either.

For women, the right size, curve and consistency is at least as important as it is for men. If breasts are over-sized and pendulant, this can contribute to a self image as destructive as a bad facial scar. Non-existent breasts can cause as much misery—so, incidentally, can a pair that don't match. **Something** can always be done.

The man who has poorly developed chest muscles can hardly expect his bones to do it all. With chest exercise to keep muscles flexible plus weight lifting to give them bulk and definition and endurance exercise to expand his lungs, he can expect the very most. If he had once been muscular and gave up exercise, he probably has a "breast problem" some flat-chested women wish they had, but on him it looks grotesque. Repair calls for diet to get rid of the deposits of fats, plus the right exercises.

For the woman who wants more of a line, the answer is fairly simple even if it does mean work. Have you seen those pictures of weight lifters who look as though they need a 36C brassiere? They have not developed breast glands, of course, but the pectoral muscles which lie (even in women) **under** the breast. The answer, since you cannot increase a breast with exercise, is to build the pectorals which will then push out and lift up the breasts you have.

For the woman who has too much of a good thing, there are two thoughts. If the excess is **fat,** as you lose weight and improve muscle tone, there ought to be less of it. In time even the shape will improve if you continue your exercises.

However, if these glands are the cause of deep distress then you've got to make a decision. If the size and shape of your breasts disturb you seriously enough to affect your happiness and your image of yourself, then the answer is plastic surgery. This can do almost anything you want, build up, take away, or make both breasts even in size and shape. The days when such operations were taboo are long gone and now it is accepted that a woman's figure can disfigure her emotionally. But before you undertake such a project make sure that exercise won't save you the expense. Give a conscientious exercise program six months, keeping track of progress by careful measurement. If it hasn't worked for you, then consider surgery. (Incidentally, there's nothing says a man can't have an operation if his skin refuses to snap back after the same six-month period.)

CHEST AND BUST LINE TIPS

- *To make a "puny" chest wide and muscular, lift weights, do exercises 92 and 93.*
- *To improve size and function, do endurance work, do exercises 96-103.*
- *To improve chest muscle flexibility and to improve posture, do exercises 26, 27, 30.*
- *To take up slack and improve muscle tone, do exercises 28 and 29.*
- *To build a larger bust, do exercises 92 and 93.*
- *To even out unequal sides, do exercise 92 with the arm of the smaller side.*
- *To slim an oversized bustline if the rest of you is oversized, do most of the exercises in this book and consider the diet on page 154. Do 31 often.*

ARM STRENGTH

How often arms give away a person's age! If you are a man and have used your arms well and vigorously, they will be smooth and well muscled. If you are not damaged by tension you can separate each muscle out with your fingers when the arm is relaxed. A muscle in good shape is **never** stiff and hard when relaxed. (If yours are stiff and hard have a good masseur go to work on them; you have tension-caused **fibrositis**.)

If you are a woman and have been vigorous and active, it will show in slender smooth arms without any sag underneath. If you have been fat and lost weight but not troubled to repair muscle tone, you will have an empty, swinging sack under each arm. If you are under considerable tension your arms may be heavy, but that isn't fat alone. That's also "fibrositis," the thickening of tissue. Pinch the outside of your arm. Does it hurt? That's fibrositis. Take hold of the flesh at the back of the upper arm . . . is there a hard lumpy quality? That's fibrositis.

What will improve a woman's arms? Exercise. And don't worry about getting "muscles." The muscles will be there to form the curves. Just remember those Russian girl gymnasts. Their arms are like steel, yet they look like Dresden china.

Men should remember that while it is universally accepted that men look at women, women look at men, and one of the first things they look for is muscle.

ARM STRENGTH TIPS

- *Exercise will not build unsightly muscles on girls. Arms will grow stronger, but it will show only in better tone and smooth curved lines.*
- *Exercise will put observable muscles on boys and men. Isometrics which build for power only (exercises 81-85) must be offset by free exercises* **26** *and* **27**.
- *The best arm exercise is still the push up, exercise* **28**, *but do it as described, not in the incomplete fashion when they are half done, but fast.*
- *Isotonics (weight lifting) are the surest builder of arm muscles. Do exercises* **87, 88, 89, 91, 92, 93**, *gradually increasing the weights.*
- *Fibrositis caused by tension often mars arms. Use the same type of pinching massage described in exercise* **64e** *and then do exercises* **22** *and* **23**.

CHEST AND BUSTLINE   Also Arm Strength

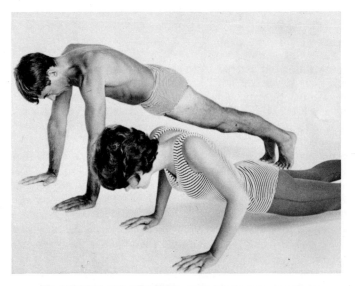

28 PUSH-UPS AND LET-DOWNS Start (whether you can do a push-up or not) at top of push-up. Keeping body absolutely rigid, lower slowly taking five full seconds to reach a resting place on floor. Last three inches will be the worst. When you touch down swing both arms around so that hands touch high above waist. Again, push up **SLOWLY**, taking three full seconds. Do half your optimum number in test #9 twice daily.

If you can't even do one, use spread-leg position, which takes some of the weight off your arms. Lower slowly to resting position and get back up any way you can. Do five such let-downs night and morning. Within a short time you will be able to push up at least once.

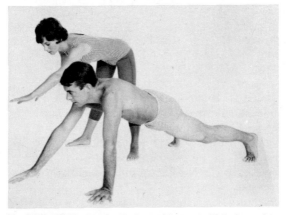

29 HAND WALK Start with feet wide apart. Walk forward on hands (without bending knees) until you are at full stretch. This should take three hand steps in three counts. On fourth count, let your body droop as in **exercise 30** below. On counts "five" and "six," take two hand-walk steps back, and on "seven" and "eight" push erect. Do eight.

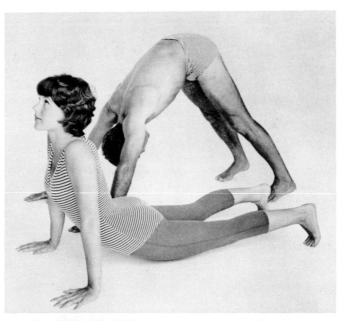

30 EXTEND AND TUCK Start resting on hands with body at full stretch, head up, feet facing straight forward (not turned out). Without moving hands or feet, press back up, forcing heels flat to floor as you press head down hard between arms. Do eight.

WAISTLINE AND MIDRIFF

A thick waist and a rubbery midriff, or a "pot," by any other name would still be unattractive, difficult to clothe and impossible to explain, since they are never seen on healthy, attractive people.

Not only does excess weight at the waist mar your appearance, it also interferes with sport and romance. In the first case, a fat, stiff mid-section is hard to handle in bending and twisting. In the second, who would look twice?

The only activity left to many these days is walking (and not much of that) and while walking does improve legs, circulation and over-all condition, it does very little for the area under consideration. Sitting, our major occupation, does a great deal, however—all of it bad.

Get rid of a "pot?" There is no such thing as "spot reducing" if you mean doing nothing about all of you while doing something for one small part of you. There is such a thing as spot reducing if you mean doing something about all of you—and something special for one part of you. To get that waist and midriff back in line, consult the diet (*page* **154**) and Exercise 64c under **"fibrositis."** Then spend plenty of time with the specific exercises for this area.

WAISTLINE AND MIDRIFF TIPS

- *Spot reduction, if you try to work just one spot, won't work.*
- *If you give extra work to a specific area while doing all you can to cut down on calories and increase circulation and muscle tone with a general program, spot reduction will work.*
- *The waist and midriff are two places where fat shows up first.*
- *Massage will help. Check exercise **64c**.*
- *Tie waist exercises into habits, such as going to the washroom, or changing tasks. Do exercise **31** often throughout the day. No fat can stay in a place that is being twisted 500 times a day.*
- *The ability to separate the upper from the lower body is a must for coordination in sport. Use exercise **32** whenever possible; always in the locker room before a game.*
- *If there's a roll over the top of your trunks get rid of it.*

WAISTLINE AND MID-RIFF EXERCISES

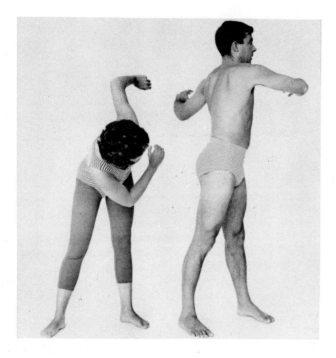

31 WAIST TWIST Start erect, legs spread wide, bent elbows at shoulder level. Twist upper body all the way to left, then way to the right. Alternate sides for sixteen counts. Next, bend forward from hips and pretend there is a small dwarf in front of you. Without moving head or hips, hit him in the head. Do sixteen, then repeat with the erect twist, followed by another bent twist series. Alternate this with exercise **32** below.

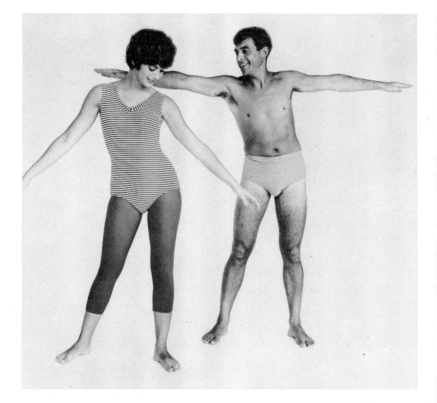

32 HIP & SHOULDER SHIFT Do this exercise in front of a table at the beginning. Stand with hands resting on it to help you stabilize upper body. Without moving shoulders or bending knees, shift hips to left. Then shift to right. Do to a quick rhythm and you will find you can move further and further to the sides. Do sixteen.

Next, press lower body against table to stabilize yourself. Stand with arms outspread and imagine you are in a closet. There is a six-inch space from each hand to the wall. Without moving hips or tilting wings, reach to the right as if to touch that wall, then reach to the left. Do sixteen and alternate with the HIP SHIFT. Alternate this series with waist twist above.

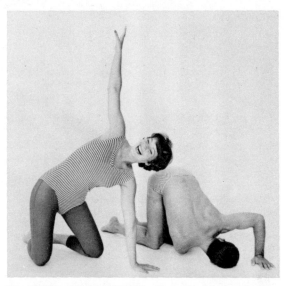

33 THREAD NEEDLE KNEELING To begin, kneel with knees apart. Fling right arm up and follow its path with head and eyes. Next, twist downward to thrust same arm into space between left hand and left knee. Try to touch floor with right ear and shoulder. Do eight and alternate for eight with the other arm. Do four series.

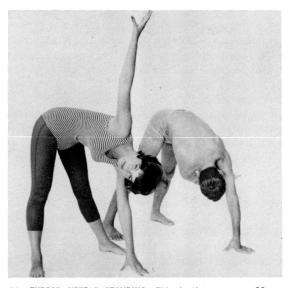

34 THREAD NEEDLE STANDING This is the same as **33** except that you are standing. (Be sure weight is on the supporting arm; some people try to fake it).

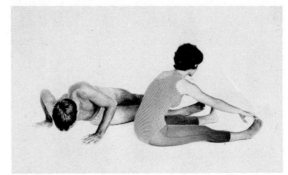

35 FLOOR DROP TOE TOUCH Sit spread-legged with back straight. Keep head and chest up. Twist upper body to the right and drop to floor, catching yourself on both hands. Push back to sitting position, and as you swing forward and towards the left for the second drop, try to touch your toes in passing. **Don't bend your knees.** Drop to left and alternate to right for eight.

HIPS

The size, shape and consistency of her hips will tell you a lot about a woman. Healthy tissue is firm and smooth. If hips look like "nervous pudding" they are soft and mushy. If they look like cement in a barrel, that's usually only "nervous pudding" in a girdle. Girdles don't hide a thing, you know, they just move it around a little.

Some women's hips are all but non-existent, and that usually means that the person is inactive even though thin. Sometimes a bit too much (if it is at least shapely) is better than nothing at all.

A seat should be firm, smooth and curved (on men and boys too). When that is the case you know there is muscle instead of fat. Muscle can only be built in a seat through action. Whether that action be sport, dance or an active occupation, it pays off in many ways. Clothes fit better, bathing suits look better, you move better, feel better and are rarely in danger of backache.

Hips answer to three things: Diet, massage and exercise. They can **always** be made more shapely, slimmer and firmer. You can **always** lose inches from the hips or seat—or you can put them on. To lose, you must diet as well as exercise and have the area loosened up through massage. If you want to put on muscle to give yourself more form, you will not need diet or massage, but you will need a great deal of hip exercise, preferably with weights.

HIP TIPS

- *Hips should be firm, smooth and curved, both men and women.*
- *Hips are another fibrositic or tension area, particularly with women. Add 64d.*
- *If there are "Saddle Bags" (hips one in measurements), do exercise 38.*
- *Heavy hips throw bodies out of line and contribute to backache. Do exercise 37.*
- *Walking (and running) will augment any program; climb stairs.*
- *Add exercises 13b and 13f to any hip reduction program.*
- *Narrow hips (side-to-side width) are desirable for men—they make shoulders look wider. But thin hips (the seat area) that are flat and unmuscled indicate weakness and inadequacy. The seat should be strong and flexible—and therefore slightly curved.*
- *If you are thin, don't be afraid you will lose. Exercise will augment the size of any muscle.*

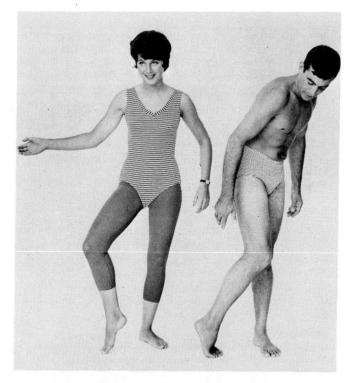

36 HIP ROTATION (Best done to "twist" music.) Stand on one foot and turn other foot in as far as possible, trying to lift the hip at the waist. Then turn foot all the way out. You will feel this on inside of thigh. Start slowly, being sure to twist as far as possible in both directions. Do eight to each side, then eight more double time.

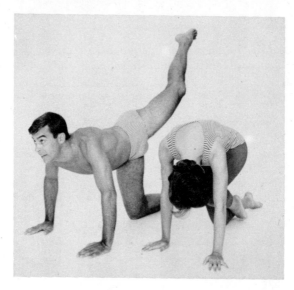

37 KNEE-TO-NOSE KICK Start kneeling. Keep arms straight.
Bring left knee as close to nose as possible (watch out that
you don't connect). Now, extend leg back and upward and at
same time lift your head. Do eight with each leg for a series.
Start with two series, work up to six. To make more difficult
hang weight bags on your ankles.

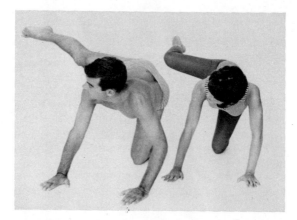

38 HYDRANT Kneel on all fours. Keeping right knee bent at
exactly same angle as for kneeling, lift leg up high to the
side. Maintain that elevation while you straighten leg out.
Feel the pull in the seat muscles and hip joint. Return leg to
its bent-knee position, still keeping it elevated. To rest the
straining muscles do not return bent leg to rest on floor, but
extend it straight backward instead, as you did in Exercise **37**.
Do "Hydrant" three times with one leg, then three with the
other. Those six repetitions make up a series. Start with two
and gradually increase until you can do six series.

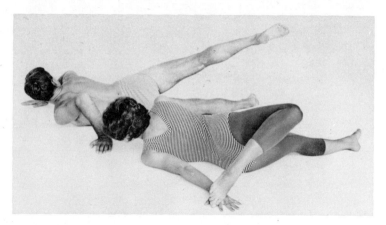

39 THE CORKSCREW Lie face down with hands at shoulder level at least 12″ out to each side. Spread legs wide. Raise the straight right leg and swing it across so that foot touches (hopefully) the left hand. DON'T MOVE THAT HAND . . . in time, the foot will reach all the way. Return to face down spread-legged position and repeat to other side. Alternate for four.

THIGHS

Heavy thighs are not caused by muscle. The only time muscle is bulbous is when it has been improperly acquired or purposely acquired for a special purpose such as heavy weight lifting—although all weight lifting does not come under the same heading (*see page* **122**). Heavy thighs are usually a combination of **fibrositis** (*page* **104**) and fat. This is particularly true when part of the body is of the proper weight, size and consistency and the hips and thighs are heavy, pneumatic and the flesh is tender when pinched (*page* **107**). In the event that **fibrositis** is present, you can assume that an excess of tension is also present . . . in excess of the physical outlet available.

The correction for this most unpleasant problem depends on 1) diet to get rid of fat and prevent the accumulation of more (*page* **154**); 2) fibrositis massage (*page* **107**) to break up the thickened tissue where the fat is trapped; 3) specific exercises for the thighs as well as other exercises to tone up the body in general; and 4) study of the causes of stress in your life. Sit down and figure out what's doing it and find ways to change things as they are. Do more physical things; go out and find some good old-fashioned fun.

THIGH TIPS

- *Muscle does not cause big thighs except in weight lifters who* want *huge thighs.*
- *Fat plus tension, which causes fibrositis (see exercise **64e**), cause big thighs.*
- *If the flesh on your thigh is thick, you have fibrositis. If, when you pinch it (64e) the flesh "dimples" and is tender, you have it. Diet will not be enough. If you just diet you will lose from face, bust and midriff, but the thighs will remain as they are. It takes diet, massage (64e) and thigh exercises 40, **41** and **42**.*
- *Fibrositis wherever it shows up, is caused by tension. Realize that you are under stress and need more physical outlet for that stress.*
- *Take up sports that you enjoy, but try to find the kind that takes you away from snack bars and food baskets—or at least provide enough activity to balance out the snack, supper or lunch.*
- *Walking, jogging, jumping rope, skiing, tennis and swimming with a kick board are all excellent.*

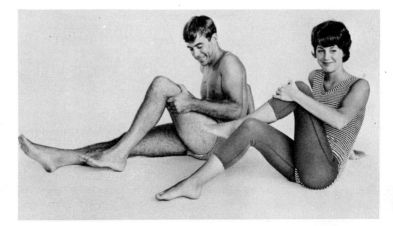

40 THIGH LIFT & CROSS If you are in very poor condition and have to start way back (bed or wheel chair—also check with chair exercises **63a, b, c,**) sit on floor, chair or bed. With the help of one or both hands, lift the thigh then take away the supporting hands and try to hold for three seconds. Increase the hold as strength increases.

Next, with hand help, draw one leg over the other knee to cross legs. With help, uncross and rest. Little by little give less and less help. Alternate for four . . . often.

If there's nothing wrong with your legs, instead of merely crossing your legs when you're sitting, make it pay off. Cross one leg over the other and then keep pushing the leg even further before bringing it to rest. You will feel strain at first around the top of the thigh and in the hip. Make a habit of this and you will be doing hip and thigh exercises all day long.

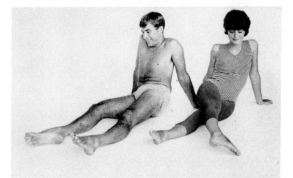

41 SPREAD-LEG CROSSOVER Sit spread-legged. Lift one leg over the other and twist it so that the big toe is leading. Cross way over and touch the big toe to the floor. Keeping the leg crossed over, rotate the foot so that your toes point to the ceiling. Then with the little toe leading cross back and **try** to rotate the leg out far enough so that the little toe touches the floor. Hold the wide leg position and rotate the foot inward so that the toes point again to the ceiling. Do four with each leg for a series. Do four series.

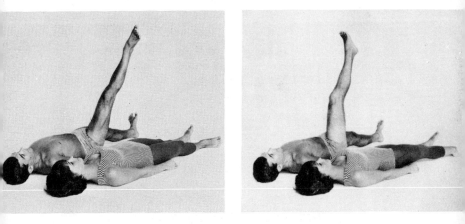

42 LEG-LIFT ROTATIONS Lie supine legs together. Rotate the right foot outward until the side is flat on the floor. Keep the leg in the outward position and raise it until it is at right angles to your body.

With the leg in the verticle position, rotate the foot inward and lower the leg to touch (but not rest on) the floor. Raise it immediately, still turned in. At the top of the lift, rotate the foot outward and lower to the starting position. Do this slowly and completely. Do four with each leg for a series. Do four series.

LEGS

There are several common problems concerning legs, the most prevalent of which is **weakness.** There are several reasons for weakness. If you have been injured or ill, walking and weight bearing are **not** the best ways to get back in the swing. While you're still in bed do the **limbering series** on pages **35** through **37,** then the **chair series** on pages **100** through **103.**

If your legs are weak because you don't use them, that's something else again. Exercise will assuredly help.

Aging brings on leg problems. As people grow older they get an ache here and a pain there. Rather than work their way through pain to make the joints and members function properly, older people try to protect themselves from pain by using each ailing area less. This leads to less and less ability to use it at all. The end is crippling. All joints should be put through full range every day even when they creak.

Varicose veins are another leg problem. They are hereditary and affect both sexes. You can't prevent them but you can do a lot about them. Better than any elastic stockings are strong resilient muscles; keep yours that way. Then, if the time ever comes when the veins must be "stripped" (removed) your legs will quickly recover and your doctor will be most grateful for giving him strong legs in good condition.

If you are fat and your legs are fat, you can correct that with diet plus exercise. However, if part of you is slender and your legs are heavy, you can figure on fibrositis. That calls not only for diet and exercise, but for massage as well, (*see page* **104** and do Exercises **40–42, 64e.** Knees and Ankles are discussed on *pages* **78** and **86.** Feet are discussed on *pages* **93** and **94.**)

LEG TIPS

- *Fat legs are not hereditary. Fat will come off the legs just as it comes off everywhere else—with diet, massage and exercise.*
  Do exercises 37, 38, 39, 42, 43, 44, 45, 46, 47, 50, 54, 56, 95-103.
- *Leg cramps often come when you are under tension and under-exercised. Try taking a quiet walk before bedtime, and do exercises on pages* **114** *through* **117.**
- *Massage before bed.*
- *Muscle will make thin legs look more attractive. Do exercises* **95 a-b.**
- *Flexibility is a must. Do exercises* **67, 73, 74.**
- *Legs do not weaken with age because they are "supposed" to, but because we don't use them enough or properly.*
- *Arteriosclerosis can affect leg action (check the section on the heart).*
- *After prolonged illness or injury don't start walking at once. Do leg exercises 43-46 and knee exercises 47-49 and even foot exercises 62a-e in bed before you get up.*
- *Varicose veins cannot be prevented, but they can be helped with*

strong elastic exercises and "flushing exercises." (See the section on knees.)

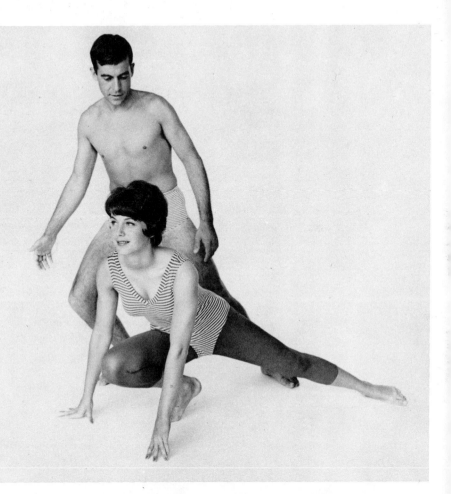

43 SPREAD-LEG WEIGHT SHIFT Stand with legs spread **wide,** feet turned slightly out. Keeping heels flat on floor and left leg absolutely straight, bend right knee far enough so that when you look down it has hidden your toes from sight. This is called a "half knee bend," or half of a full knee bend in which you would go all the way down. As you look down over your knee you should not see your foot at all and particularly not under the outside of your knee. If you do you will know that your foot is rolled over onto its inside edge, which is bad for both knee and foot. **Keep foot directly under knee.** Return to straight-leg position and repeat to left. Alternate for eight.

Next do **Weight Shift** on one level. Start with half knee bend to the right by bending right knee and keeping left knee straight. Then keeping body on exact same low level, shift weight to other side by bending left knee as you cross over. When you arrive at left side, see that right leg is then absolutely straight. Do eight.

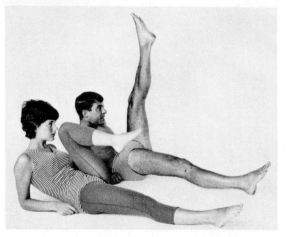

44 KNEE TO NOSE EXTEND Lie supine resting on elbows. Draw right leg in bringing knee as close to nose as possible. KEEPING THE KNEE CLOSE TO NOSE straighten leg to the vertical position. (The closer you come to your nose the better). Bend knee to knee-nose position, then stretch leg to rest on floor. Alternate for eight. (If your knee makes sounds, don't worry. Most knees rustle.)

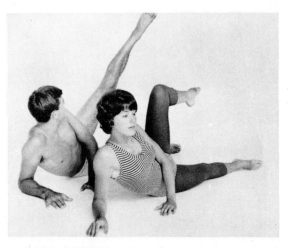

45 LATERAL EXTENSION (A note: Legs are meant to spread wide, just as they are meant to run fast in the wind, climb high on a mountain—and carry you where you want to go.)

Lie on your right side (be sure you are on your side, not lolling back on your hip.) Rest on right elbow and place left hand on floor for balance. Bring left knee to the side and up into position **behind** your left shoulder. Then extend leg outward and **up** as far as you can. Return it to the near-shoulder position, then to the starting point. Do four, then roll over to the other side for four more. This is one series. Do four.

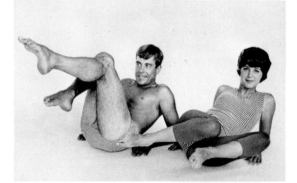

46 BICYCLE Lie supine with weight on elbows. Start exercise with "bicycle action". Do eight. Do them slowly and to full range in large circles. Then keeping **both** elbows fast to floor, which will work your waist, roll over onto your left hip and do eight more. Repeat this on the other hip. You will notice while you are "biking" on one hip or the other, it is getting a massage as your muscles work against the ungiving surface of the floor—excellent for fibrositic "saddlebags."

If you are in good shape you may want to add NO HANDS bike. Just sit up as in **Exercise 9,** but instead of tapping your feet, repeat the "bicycle" exercise without aid of an elbow rest.

KNEES

Due partially to the fact that two of our national games, football and basketball, are knee wreckers, knees have become a serious problem. Why is this when, for Europe, soccer has not? We don't build leg strength when we should—between birth and 12. If we had to walk to get where we wanted to go, we would build the legs we needed for sport (and for such difficulties as war). It is contact sports indulged in by youngsters who have never been prepared for contact sports, either by their way of life or by proper **all-year-round** coaching and calisthenics, that cause most of the knee injuries, back injuries, shoulder separations, and a host of other sports injuries.

If you have hurt a knee or if your knees are weak, there is no protection against further or future injury like strong, ever-**flexible** muscle. You can't buy it for your team, for yourself or your son. But you **can** build it. You build a muscle by "overloading" it. For example you find that with great difficulty you can do **one** deep knee bend. However, after one week of doing one at a time you find two not impossible. When you've done two every night for a week, you feel that four might not be beyond reach. So day after day, week after week you keep adding, and gradually you work yourself into the big time. That's "overloading," and it's the only way to keep improving.

So, either because you didn't know, or the coach didn't know . . . or you just plain ran into bad luck, you've got a "bad knee." Are you going to quit? You may not play football any more, but there are a dozen other sports waiting. What about tennis? That doesn't take a team. And skiing? Now **there's** a sport! What about rock climbing and mountaineering and skating and water skiing? Life's just begun. If you've got a bad knee, get after it. Yes, it may take an operation, but then again it may not. The knees are controlled mostly by muscles in the thighs called the **quadriceps.** If you put those in real order the knees may go along with you. In any case, if exercise doesn't solve the problem, there isn't a doctor in the world who won't be glad to see you strengthen both your lower legs and your "quads." It almost assures him of a successful result if a knee operation (usually a **miniscus**) is necessary. Either way, get at it.

The same exercises improve "old" knees too, and the kind that complain when the weather changes.

KNEE TIPS

- *Knees get "old" when they are not used properly and enough.*
- *Contact sports played by youngsters not trained long enough and hard enough, and not specifically enough, cause hidden knee injuries.*
- *Deep knee bends* help *weak knees, they do not hinder. Do exercises* **50,** *51, 52, 53, 54.*
- *Be sure to work a knee weakened by injury until it is as strong as the other one before going back to any "spike" sport such as tennis or skiing. Do exercise* **47.** *A pampered knee will soon cause an aching hip, you can't afford to ignore it.*
- *Knee flexibility is just as important as leg strength. Do exercises* **48** *and* **49.**
- *Poor mechanics in the foot contribute to knee problems. See page 93.*

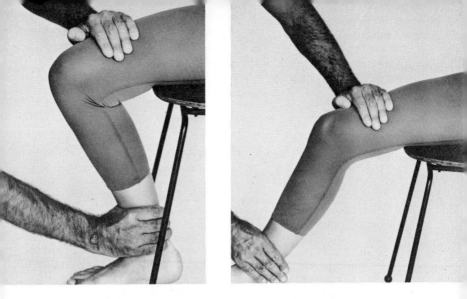

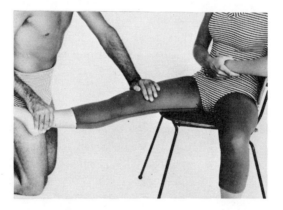

47 KNEE RESISTANCE Resistance can be had in many forms, but the best is that offered by a sensitive human being. A knee (and any other joint) will have its stronger and its weaker areas. If weights are used the resistance will either suit the weak area and underwork the strong or suit the strong and be too much for the weak. When someone else's muscle is matched with yours, the proper pressure is put on each area.

Sit on chair or table. The knee is stabilized by a hand holding it steady; resistance will be applied to the ankle. Object is to move from bent-knee to straight-leg position against that resistance. The first third of the way the leg is weak; **light resistance.** The second third the leg is much stronger; **increase the resistance.** The last third it will be weak again; **lessen the resistance.** At full stretch, tighten the thigh muscles (quadriceps) and hold for a slow count of three, then relax. Do ten. Do not make the resistance too heavy at first or the leg will tire too fast.

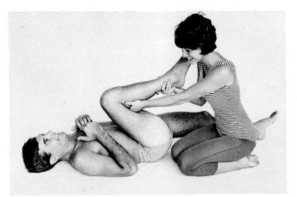

48 PASSIVE STRETCH Exerciser takes leg to be worked in hands and works it **slowly** from full stretch to bent- knee position without any help from its owner. Set up a rhythm.

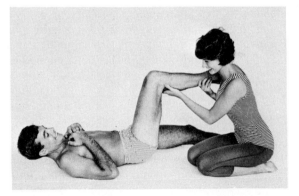

49 ACTIVE RESISTANCE This time the leg muscles resist all the way. As leg is **pulled** by its owner into bent-knee position, resistance is put on it by pulling against calf muscle and heel. At the bent-knee position exerciser places heel against her shoulder and leg is **pushed** against her resistance. Start with very gentle resistance and gradually increase. Work 10 minutes, or less if leg tires.

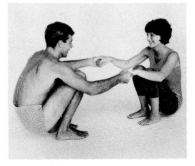

50 FLAT-FOOT KNEE BENDS Except in prenatal knee bends **(Exercise 108)**, knee bends are done with knees together. Grasp hands and drop slowly into a deep knee bend with heels flat on the floor. (To do this alone, hold onto the two handles of an open door with the edge facing you.) Start with four.

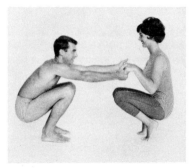

51 ALTERNATE TOE & FLAT-FOOT KNEE BENDS Just going up and down can be dull, so liven it up. One partner goes down flat-footed, which works the front muscles of the lower leg while the other partner goes down on the toes, which works arch of foot. Alternate for four.

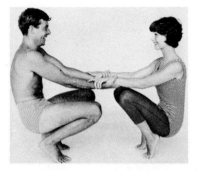

52 TOE-RISE KNEE BENDS Rise first to the toes, then slowly drop into a deep knee bend. Return to the toe-rise standing position, and end with the heels flat on the floor.

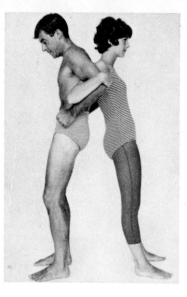

53 BACK-TO-BACK KNEE BENDS Stand back-to-back with about 2½ feet of space between the two pairs of heels (you may need more; the first descent will tell you how much space). Lock arms and, leaning against each other, go slowly down into a deep knee bend. Rest in the sitting position for a count of three and return to a standing position. Do four.

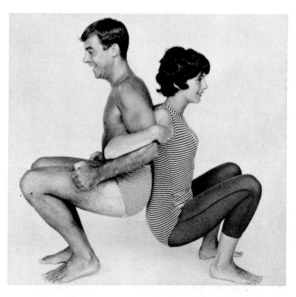

RESISTANCE AND BALANCE

The dictionary says that **resistance** is the act of **resisting, opposing** or **withstanding** the opposition offered by one body to the pressure or movement of another—and that is exactly what resistance is in exercise. It is not the effort on the part of one person or body to **overcome** the other.

The weakest muscle can offer at least a little resistance (provided it has life at all) to even the strongest muscle, and by so doing, gain in strength. This is as true for a small boy working against his father as a woman working against a man. A balance point can always be found, wherein the weaker puts forth great effort while the stronger tempers his strength to match. One gains in strength and the other in sensitivity and control.

RESISTANCE AND BALANCE TIPS

- *Strength is not enough, you need sensitivity and control.*
- *Such control makes working with partners of unequal weight and strength possible.*
- *Strength plus flexibility in proper timing and intensity yield coordination. Balanced resistance is a lesson in intensity. Do exercises* **54** *and* **85.**

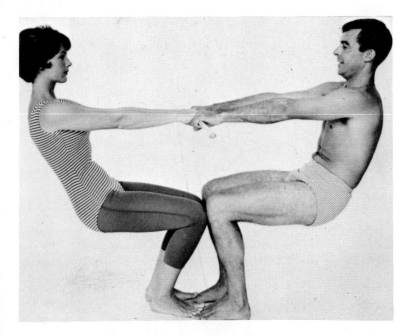

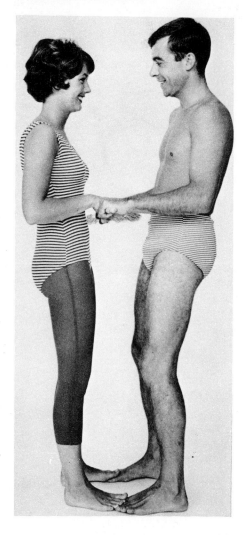

54 LEAN OUT & DOWN If the two partners lean out exactly the same distance from center, the heavier will pull the other over. Delicate balancing is the trick and the lesson. Grasp hands or the handle of a broom or mop. The **lighter** partner covers the other partner's toes. Lean out slowly to full arm stretch. Go slowly down into a deep knee bend and as slowly rise. Do this exercise to slow music. Try for four without losing balance.

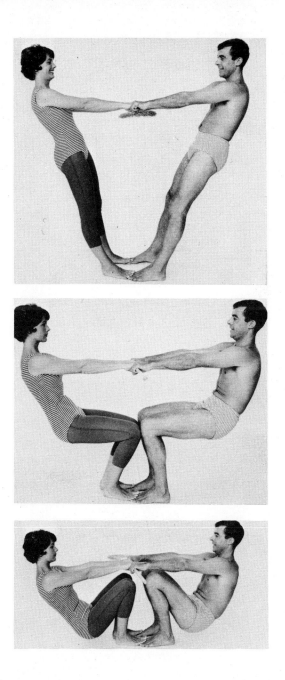

For other resistance and point of balance, see exercise 86.

ANKLES, SOLEUS, CALVES

Weak ankles, inflexible heel cords and tight hamstrings account for a great many sports injuries, a great many awkward and ungainly walks and a great deal of discomfort.

To strengthen ankles that are either weak or at some time in your life were injured and not brought back to full strength, you need resistance exercises, as well as foot exercises, massage and walking exercise. This is a must if you want to move around with ease and without fatigue. The same gentle (but growing stronger all the time) resistance is applied to ankles as well as other joints and muscles.

Tight heel cords and soleus (a muscle in the back of the lower leg) will prevent full range of motion. You can't get enough **"vorlager"** (forward lean) in skiing, or enough height in a jump after a ball. Since the muscles pull all the time, your legs tire easily.

Everyone needs flexibility in the hamstrings (muscles running down the backs of the legs from under the buttocks).

ANKLE, SOLEUS, AND CALF TIPS

- *Strong ankles rarely turn. If you have a weak ankle, strengthen it with exercises **55** and **56**.*
- *Swollen angles respond to full range of motion against resistance. Do exercise **55**.*
- *Tight foot and lower leg muscles often cause leg cramps—stretch them with exercise **56**.*
- *Unattractive straight-line calves can be given curves. Do exercises 50-54 and **56**.*
- *For any sport requiring the use of legs, stretch the soleus with exercise **56b**.*
- *Poor foot mechanics contribute to shaky ankles. See page **xx**.*

55 ANKLE RESISTANCE The ankle is to be put through "full range of motion" at first "passively" with the exerciser doing all the work and the ankle completely relaxed. Look at **62a** for what is called "extending", in which the instep is stretched and the toe pointed down, then look at **62b** for "flexing," in which the front of the foot is drawn up. Do several of these to set the pattern. Next rotate the foot inward a little, then outward.

A pattern of movement is set; now add resistance. Your exerciser (the girl in the pictures) holds the back of your foot and places her fist on the ball of your foot. Your foot, pressing against her fist, is then 'extended". Don't let her make the fist's resistance too hard for you to work through. Next, still holding the back of the foot, your exerciser places a hand over your lower foot. You then pull your foot upward against this resistance. Make sure it is the ankle and no other part of the leg that is doing the work. Do four such movements, then shake the foot loose to relax it.

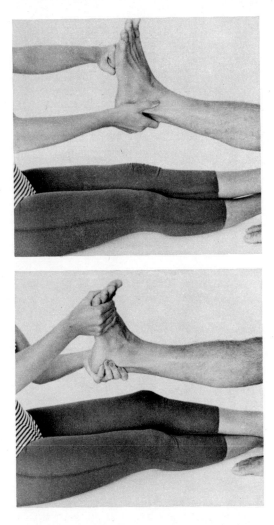

Still holding the back of your foot, exerciser places the fingers of her free hand against the inside of the front of your foot; you press the foot inward against her resistance. Finally, she places a hand against the outside of the front of the foot and you press outward against resistance. Do four and shake loose to relax.

To strengthen a weak ankle or prepare for a sport, do this exercise several times daily.

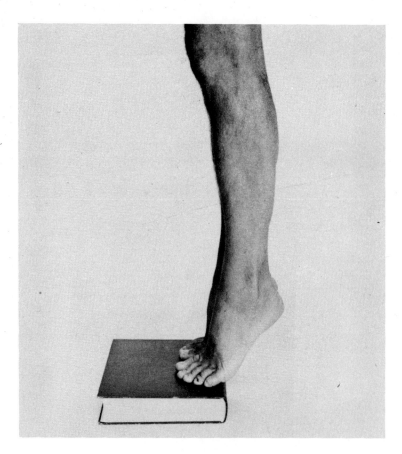

56a HEEL CORD AND SOLEUS STRETCH Stand with balls of feet on a book. If your balance is precarious hold onto a table. Start by standing on toes, then let yourself down slowly until heels touch floor. If heel cords and soleus are sc tight that heels cannot touch, do a few little bounces downward, then go up to toe-rise position. Do four. If heels **can** touch the floor, do this exercise a few times, then add a book. Use the bouncing technique to stretch the muscles several times daily.

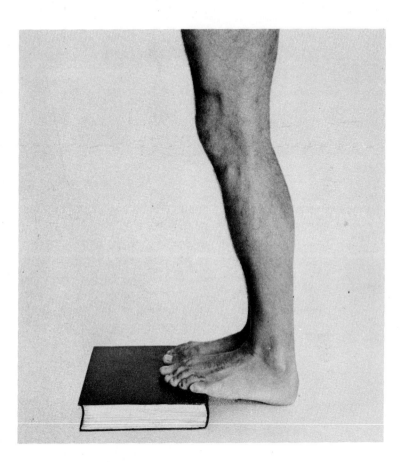

56b CALF STRENGTHENER To improve strength and appearance of calf do same exercise as above but carry increasingly heavy weights in both hands (two loaded suitcases will do nicely). Add weight to suitcases as strength improves; use thicker books under your feet as stretch improves. Do slowly.

To relax backs of ankles after the exercise, do **62e**.

WRISTS AND HANDS

Wrists, hands and even fingers don't seem very important until some part of them stops working properly. If you lack hand strength you may not discover it until you need the ultimate in strength in a life and death crisis. Then there's **arthritis;** you are certainly aware of it when **that** attacks you, but when the doctor says exercise, do you know what exercise?

Weak wrists make poor golf scores; you may even notice pain when you type, paint the ceiling or wring out socks.

As with every other part of the body, hand exercise is important. It can even give you that handshake known as warm and firm.

WRIST AND HAND TIPS

- *Don't be satisfied with any weak area; you never know when you will need it.*
- *To improve any manual dexterity (including typing speed) improve strength. Do exercise* **58.**
- *When the doctor says exercise your arthritic fingers, he means it, even if it hurts. Do exercise* **58.**
- *To improve golf scores, exercise wrists against resistance. Do exercise* **57.**
- *To relax hands that tend to fidget, do exercise* **58** *until your hands are exhausted, then relax.*

WRISTS

While it is usually more stimulating to have company, this exercise can also be done alone.

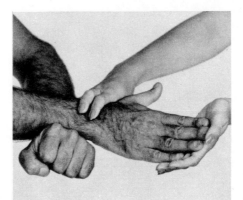

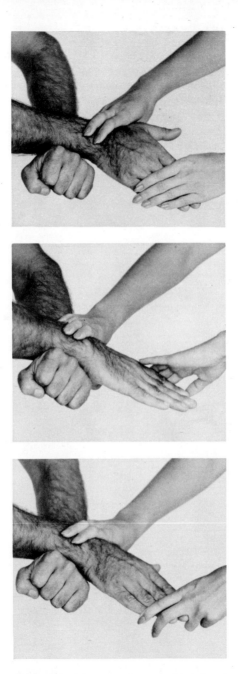

WRIST RESISTANCE Stabilize weak wrist on table or against other hand. a) Press "good" hand ⌄wnward against gentle resistance from the wrist, not just from the fingers. b) Press hand upward ⌐ainst resistance. c) Rotate hand inward against resistance of fingers placed against thumb side ⌐d outward against resistance from outer side. Spend three or four minutes on this exercise several ⌐es a day.

HANDS

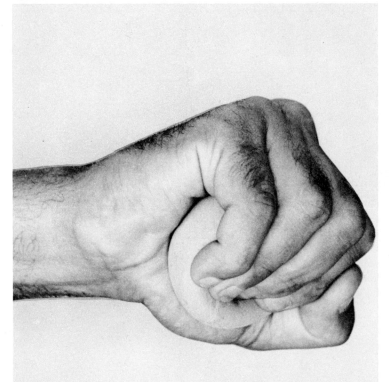

58 SQUEEZE You can squeeze a fairly soft ball a little or you can squeeze it a lot. You can put a little pressure on it, or you can almost rupture it. Whatever shape your hands are in, this exercise can help. If for any reason you have been bed ridden, seriously ill, badly hurt, the SQUEEZE will help. It may be your first effort to get back into shape—after a heart attack, for instance. When you squeeze anyhing you use your hand, wrist, even your arm muscles, and you improve the circulation in your entire arm.

Squeeze and hold for slow count of five, then relax. The more you work, the better will be your results.

FEET

Most babies are born with good feet but by the time they reach age 20 most are having some sort of foot trouble. Some of such trouble is due to shoes, some to tight socks and stockings, but most of it is due to the fact that we don't walk, run, jump and climb enough.

Flat feet, once thought to be sufficiently disabling to keep a man out of the army, are now so common that if we excluded their owners, we'd have no army. Corns, calluses and other disfiguring results of incorrect footwear are the usual, and it is a rare foot that is free of them or of ingrown toenails and bunions.

Not content with their own misery, feet cause a host of ills to other parts of the body. There is a type of foot known as "The Classical Greek Foot" and you will find it on almost every statue carved in that era You may also find it on yourself. If your second toe is longer than your big toe . . . feel "classical," but also warned. A foot with good mechanics is an excellent support which means it supports you without undue effort. It is like a tripod and the three points of support are your heel, the first joint of the big toe in the ball of your foot . . . and the outside of the foot at the first joint of the little toe. With such a foot you can walk without a wobbly ankle which in turn wears your knees and ultimately your hips. You can balance well in dance and sports. You have an advantage. That "Classical Greek Foot" with its long second toe is not a tripod, it is a knife edge. The weight moves from your heel straight forward into the first joint of that second toe which is almost the center of the front of your foot. You spend your life trying to stay up on that edge which is easiest done barefoot or in sandals. (That's how the Greeks handled it.) The shoe wearer however gets a callous under the ball of the foot and then in an effort to relieve the pressure from a so-called "fallen arch," pastes on a pad under the offending callous thinking to lift the arch. This compounds the problem. The second toe, already taking to itself the job the toe is too short to do, gets even more height from the pad. Frantic big toe and little toe, grabbing for balance, are soon covered with corns and even bunions can appear.

Exercise can strengthen the muscles of foot, ankle, leg, knee and hip for the owner of a long second toe, but that won't change the mechanics. However, a small ¼ inch pad of felt placed **under the ball of the foot where the first joint of the big toe rests** can give you a much more stable foot. Be very sure that it is **only under the big toe joint** and does not encroach in any way on the area occupied by the second toe. Glue the pads to the insides of your shoes and see if you don't feel more secure at once.

When you know the mechanics of your feet are right, **then** exercise them well and often. Foot massage will help too and later when you are ready for it, walk and jog on uneven trails.

No matter what shape your feet are in, if your job means standing, have several pairs of shoes on hand and keep changing. Kick off your shoes whenever you can, even when you are sitting at a desk. Sitting is bad for feet. It slows circulation, ankles swell and toes may even cramp. Put your feet up on the desk, the work table, on an ottoman —anything that brings your feet up as you lie back to rest.

FEET TIPS

- *Most poor feet are the result of disuse and misuse.*
- *Age doesn't cause poor feet, bad habits and poor shoes do.*
- *Proper shoes can only go so far to help aching feet; exercise is just as important. Do exercises* **59, 60, 61.**
- *Flat feet need not cause weakness or pain. Feet can be as flat as pancakes and still function normally if the muscle on the outside of the lower leg (Anterior Tibialis) is strong. Do exercises* **60a, 63c.**
- *When heels of shoes are worn down unevenly it indicates that ankles as well as feet are in need of strengthening. Do exercises* **55** *and* **56** *and check for the long 2nd toe.*
- *Feet must be flexible as well as strong. Do exercises 62a,* **62b,** *63a.*
- *Wearing high heels shortens heel cords and soleus. Do exercise 56.*

FOOT EXERCISES

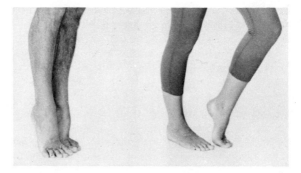

59a TOE RISES Feet parallel flat on the floor. Rise **slowly** to a count of four. Lower to four. On next rise keep same beat, but take five counts to reach the top and five to lower. On the next, six, then seven and finally eight counts. Finish off with eight quick up-and-down rises, one to a beat.

59b ALTERNATE TOE RISES Keep balls of feet and toes flat on floor. This will improve flexibility of joints where toes join your foot. Standing on one flat foot, do a toe rise with the other foot. Change feet to rhythm. Do sixteen.

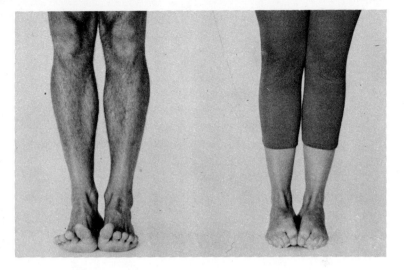

60a HOT PENNY Stand feet parallel. Raise all ten toes at once as if there were hot pennies under them. Lower. First do eight, then alternate with **60b** for another set of eight.

60b MOUSE TRAP Start with feet pressed close together. Roll to outsides of both feet and curl toes hard, be sure heels and toes are touching. Relax and repeat for eight. Then alternate with **60a** for eight.

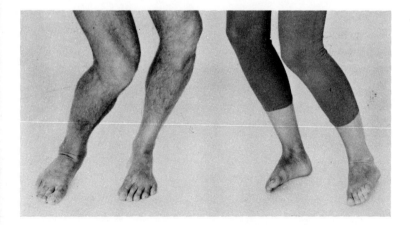

61 EDGING Stand feet parallel and a little apart. (Can also be done with feet close together). Bend both knees and, keeping the upper body still, push both knees to one side. On next count thrust them to the other side. (To make this easy at first, rest both hands on table to stabilize you.) See that your feet stay flexible and loose, rolling way over onto their sides. Do sixteen.

FOOT MASSAGE TIPS

- *Far more important than the style of your shoes is the fit.*
- *More important than shoes is keeping feet strong through exercise and supple with massage: see exercise **62**.*
- *Use a good lubricating cream often (men too).*
- *Take 10 minutes for foot massage after any sport and a few minutes before bedtime.*
- *If your feet ache and you think soaking will help, do so, but always add massage.*
- *Massage your feet before going out for the evening if they are tired.*
- *Massage improves circulation in the feet. If yours are habitually cold, spend a few minutes two or three times a day on foot massage.*

FOOT MASSAGE

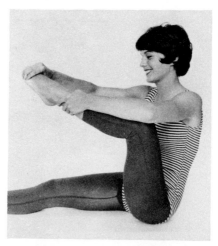

62a EXTEND Hold ankle in one hand and press down on lower instep to force an arch into your foot. If at first this causes a cramp wiggle your toes and it will go away. Hold for three, pressing a little more each count.

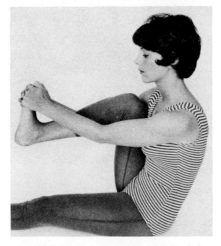

62b FLEX Place both hands on ball of foot and pull upwards to stretch bottom and back of foot, the soleus and heel cords. Hold for three, pulling a little extra on each count.

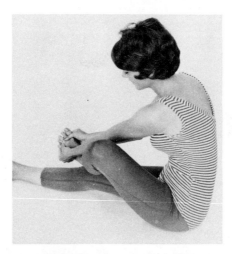

62c TOE SPREAD Your toes have been too often cramped in shoes. Spread them wide and work your fingers against the tight places in between them as if they were webs and you were trying to make longer toes.

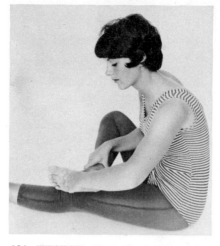

62d KNUCKLING Place the knuckle of hand against ball of foot and knead it in circles. Put as much pressure on it as you can.

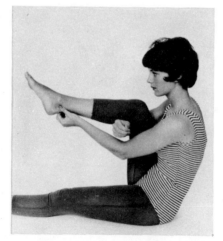

62e RELAX HEEL Take hold of heel cords down close to heel and work them from side to side moving your fingers slowly up the leg.

CHAIR EXERCISES

There are many reasons for starting your exercise program from bed or chair. You may have been ill and are on the mend. You may have had an operation. In either case remember that time in bed can take more out of you than a stretch in the salt mines. Bed is not your normal 24-hour habitat; you have lost muscle tone as well as elasticity and strength. Circulation has slowed even though your heart may beat faster. You are probably weak and the first effort will bring on a film of sweat. That's not the time to stop, it's just time to understand what's the trouble so you won't be dismayed.

To get back to life you start at the beginning, which means wiggling your toes, tightening your leg muscles as you lie there, then adding your seat muscles. Pick your head up and look at your feet, then lie back and rest. Day by day as your doctor says you may, lift your head a little higher, then add shoulders. Slide one foot up to the bent-knee position, then the other, then both. At that point add the limbering series (*see pages* **35–37**). Get a ball to squeeze (*page* **92**).

Another reason for doing "chair exercises" has nothing to do with illness . . . it's because you are stuck all day in a chair. Exercises 63a, b, c, and d can be done under anybody's desk, anybody's kitchen table, work table, dinner table. They can even be done at board meetings and nobody the wiser.

If you've had a bad break and are in a wheel chair you still must keep muscles firm and limber and your blood circulating. If you are to avoid depression, you have to be doing something constructive for yourself. Do all you can of the Exercise 63 group and as many of the limbering series Exercises 12a-e as you can manage, even it it's only 12c. Do Exercises 20 and 21 for neck and shoulder tension, 24 and 25 for shoulders, 26 and 27 for both shoulders and chest. If legs are your problem, have someone help you with Exercises 47, 48 and 55. You can do 57 and 58 without help from anybody. Be sure to have someone do foot massage for you at least once a day. Feet feel better when they are warmed that way even when you don't stand on them.

CHAIR EXERCISE TIPS

- *If you have been ill in bed you just don't get up and walk off, you prepare.*
- *Bed rest is debilitating and unless you exercise a little and get some strength back before you get up for good, you may find yourself back where you were. Do chair exercise 63 from the first minute your doctor says you may.*
- *Your feet, so long on a level with the rest of you, will swell when they are put down at first.*

- *Your circulation was sluggish while you lay still, it will need some pepping up (that's one reason people feel dizzy the first day up).*
- *If you are confined to a wheel chair, that's no reason for giving up. If you can keep your body limber and well toned even though you must sit, you will find you are not depressed and can find the strength to do what you want to do after all.*
- *Chair exercise can be done almost anywhere and at any time.*
- *The fact that so much of our time is spent sitting is the most valid reason for doing exercises in chairs. Exercises **63a-d** can be done at your desk, during homework, while you are writing letters, riding in a car, even in front of TV.*
- *Exercise **63d** can be done while you are talking on the phone.*
- *Exercise **63f** should be done every time you hang up the phone.*
- *Tie in exercise **20** for neck tension and **21** for shoulder tension.*
- *Since most of your gadgets work against you, make chairs work for you.*

CHAIR EXERCISES

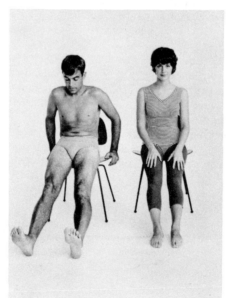

63a POINT & PULL UP (EXTEND & FLEX)
Sit on the edge of a chair and extend legs straight. Pull toes up as far as you can and hold for five counts. Then point toes sharply down and hold for five. Alternate four each way.

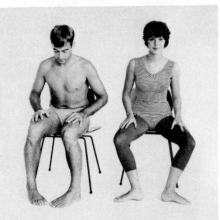

63b IN & OUT Place feet about a foot apart. Now, keeping heels on floor, swivel the toes in to touch, then all the way outward. Do eight.

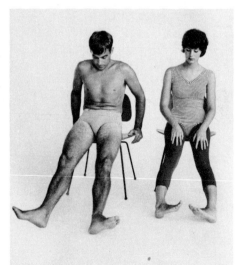

63c CIRCLES Start by pulling toes straight up as you did in **63a**. Then rotate them outward, tightening the muscles of the thighs. Follow through by pointing downward as in **63a**. Then rotate them in. Do eight complete circles.

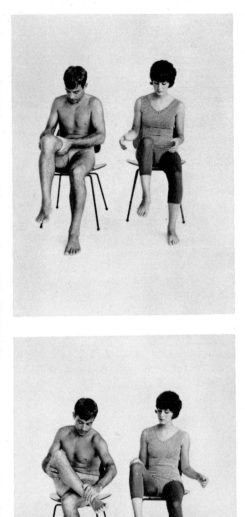

63d KNEE LIFTS Lift up one knee with one or both hands. At the top of the lift remove support and try to maintain the lift without it. Try first for one second, then two, and so on to ten. Alternate for eight. When you can lift without support, try "marching" to a good brisk beat.

63e CROSS & OPEN This calls for a chair with arms. Start with knee in crossed position even if you have to lift it there. From the knee-crossed position, swing the leg wide and drape it over the arm of the chair. Do four with each leg.

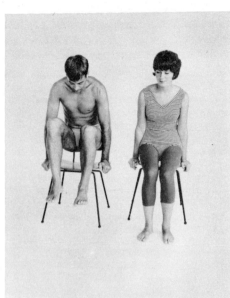

63f SEAT LIFTS If there are plans to get you out of that chair, then begin to strengthen abdominals, back, arm and shoulder muscles well before D day. Place hands on the arms of the chair or on the chair seat. Then, leaning forward, lift yourself off your seat slowly. Start with just one inch, hold for a count of three and sink back. Do this on and off all the time you are in the chair and try to hold longer each day.

The full seat lift—feet off floor—isn't easy and is to be done only after you are your old self again. Place hands on the arms of the chair or the seat and lift yourself clear. Work at a desk? Do one every time you hang up the telephone.

FIBROSITIS TIPS

- *Fibrositis is a thickening of the tissue caused by unconscious tensing of certain areas of your body when you are under stress.*
- *Typical fibrositic areas are "Dowager's Hump" (at the base of the neck), shoulders, upper arms, down the back on both sides of the spine, hips "one" (see Measurements on page 19), thighs and often the lower leg.*
- *Fibrositic tissue is very tender when pinched (see Fibrositic Massage, pages 104–107).*

FIBROSITIS MASSAGE

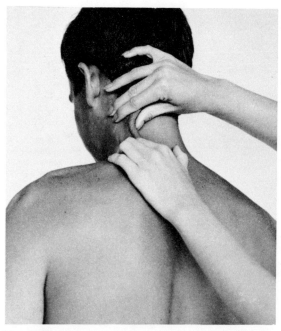

64a NECK Take the tissue between thumbs and forefingers of both hands and, starting at the base of the neck, work thumb of one hand against fingers of the other. Move hands slowly upward back and forth against the tender thick area. Go right up into the hair line on both sides of the spine. Spend at least one or two minutes every other night.

- *When pinched, the flesh "dimples"; it's hard and thick.*
- *Such thick areas are not merely fat, and if diet is tried in order to slim them, weight will come off of other areas first—and often hardly at all from the fibrositic areas.* Pinching massage *is a must to break this up.*
- *Fibrositis contributes to muscle pain in back, shoulders, neck, and is even involved in tension headaches.*

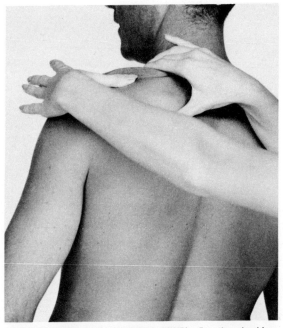

64b SHOULDERS (AND DOWAGERS HUMP) For the shoulders, start at the edge of the shoulder and work one hand against the other, right into the neck. Pinching massage is just that— it pinches, it breaks up, and it hurts. Be gentle at first. As fibrositis breaks up you will be able to be more severe.
For dowager's hump, an ugly lump just below the back of the neck, you will need strong hands, as this is particularly resistant material. Work this area very hard. (Do also Exercises **21** and **27**.)

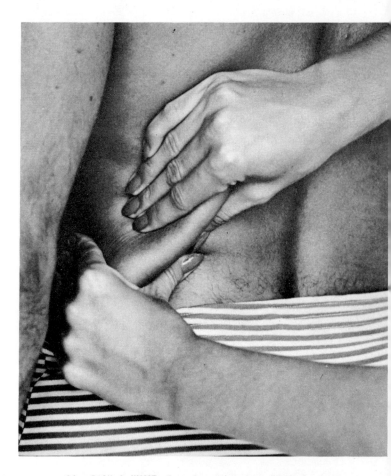

64c BACK & WAIST Best done lying down. Work one hand against the other all the way up both sides of back. A spare tire at the waist? Give an extra dose. (Do also Exercise **31**.)

TO MASSAGE ARMS, start at the elbow and work upward. There is nothing in medical literature that says you will cause any damage. A bruise might appear, but that is unimportant compared with the thick tissue which invariably mars appearance and often causes real pain. (Do also Exercise **22**.)

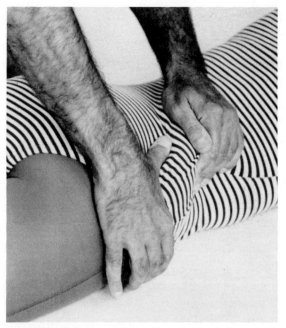

64d HIPS Hips often call for strong hands. Don't work too long in one place. A minute at any one spot is long enough. (Do also Exercises **37** and **38.**)

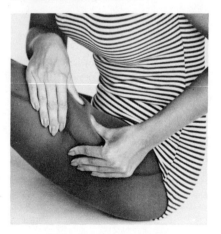

64e THIGHS As many as four inches can be removed from thighs in a matter of a few months with diet, exercise and massage. (Do also Exercises **41** and **42.**)

DOUBLES TIPS

- *Working with someone else is more fun than working alone. It can also be more difficult.*
- *Double exercises take timing and balance. The slower they are done, the more you will benefit from them.*
- *It is not necessary for both of you to be the same weight or size or to have the same strength. The trick lies in matching one body to another in intensity and timing. Exercise **65.***
- *Never hurry, never fight the action and never make a sudden unpredictable move. Try to get into a slow rhythm and stay with it. Exercise **66.***

DOUBLES EXERCISE

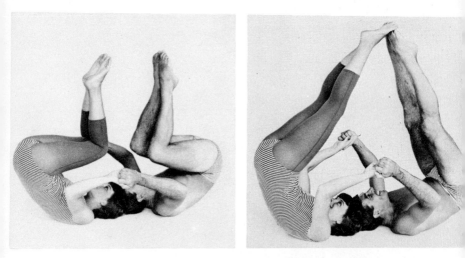

65 DOUBLE OVERHEAD PULL-UP (For abdominal strength, arm strength, and leg flexibility.) Lie supine head-to-head and holding hands. (This can also be done holding a broom stick.) Draw your knees over your heads at the same time. Gradually straighten legs until toes touch. Try to keep buttocks high off floor. To make this more difficult: when you reach the top of the pull-up, see that foot meets foot. Hold the feet against each other, legs spread wide. Close again and lower.

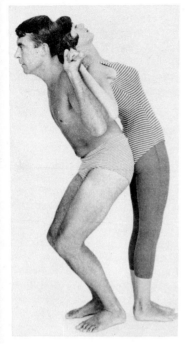

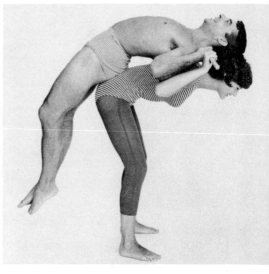

66 BACK LIFT This takes real trust and cooperation! The smaller partner will find the "lift" easier because the trick in this exercise lies in getting the seat of the lifter **under** the seat of the lifted.

Stand back-to-back, hands holding a broomstick placed just behind shoulders. Lifter stands with feet well apart for balance, knees bent to get **under** the seat of the other. Person to be lifted relaxes every muscle but hands and arms. As lifter bends slowly forward, the lifted arches the back and hangs loose and free. RELAX—IF YOU TENSE OR BRING UP YOUR LEGS OR TWIST, YOU WILL ROLL OFF TO THE SIDE. Do this to very slow music.

FLEXIBILITY TIPS

- *Strength plus* flexibility *in the proper timing and intensity yield coordination. One without the other is only half the story.*
- *Muscles not trained in flexibility cannot give up contraction and are therefore prone to fatigue.*
- *Inflexible muscles are more easily injured than flexible muscles which can stretch easily.*
- *Tense people generally have inflexible areas, namely the back and hamstrings (test* **6,** *page 13) and need a great deal of physical outlet as a balance.*
- *Flexibility exercises should* never *be done until after muscles have been warmed up (page 142).*
- *For inflexibility do exercises 26, 27, 30, 48, 49, 56 and 67–74—with 74 possibly the most important flexibility exercise of all.*

FLEXIBILITY EXERCISES

WARNING: WARM UP BEFORE DOING THESE EXERCISES. (See page 142.)

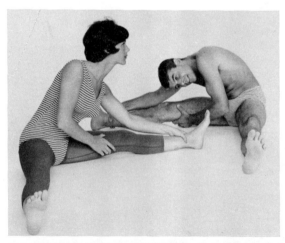

67a SPREAD-LEG STRETCH WITH HEAD UP Start sitting spread-legged with knees straight. Grasp left ankle with left hand for calf if you can't reach that far) and KEEPING YOUR READ **UP,** pull body forward as if trying to put chin on big toe. Bounce forward eight left, eight right for a series. Do four series.

67b SPREAD-LEG STRETCH WITH HEAD DOWN Now try to put your ear on your knee. LET ARMS DO PULLING. Do four series.

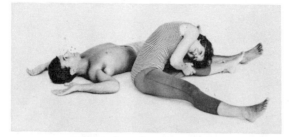

68 FLEXIBILITY ROLL OUT Sit spread-legged. Roll back, hands above head. Swing up and try to touch left ear to left knee (knees straight). Roll back and repeat, swinging up to right. Alternate for eight.

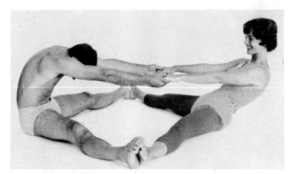

69 SEESAW Face partner with legs spread wide. Feet should touch, but if one is less flexible than the other, that one's feet may rest against the ankles of the other, more flexible, partner. Grasp hands (or if you are too inflexible to touch, grasp a bath towel). One leans back **slowly** to pull the other forward. Then the other pulls in the opposite direction. Try to be relaxed and not pull too hard. Seesaw for eight pulls.

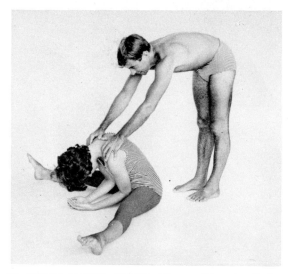

70 PASSIVE STRETCH BOUNCE Sit spread-legged, allowing upper body and head to fall forward. RELAX. Partner presses gently on shoulders in easy bounces eight times. Then sit tall to stretch and repeat. Do four.

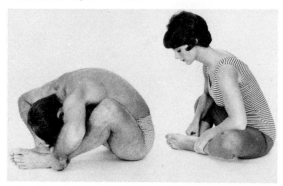

71 LOW BACK STRETCH Sit with feet drawn up close, soles pressed against each other. Grasp ankles. In easy bounces, try to draw your head down to touch toes. Eight bounces to a series. Do two series, then alternate with Exercise **72.**

72 CROTCH STRETCH Sit with feet drawn up, soles pressed against each other. Grasp ankles and let elbows rest on knees. Using ankles as anchors, press elbows down firmly on knees. Hold for three counts and release. Relax for three counts and repeat. Do eight and alternate with Exercise **71.**

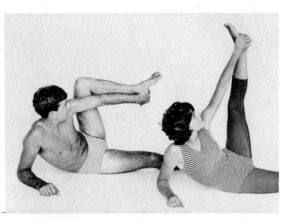

73 LEG EXTENSIONS Lie on right side resting on right elbow, right leg extended. Take instep of left foot in left hand while knee is bent. Extend leg straight up. If you are very flexible you can bend left arm more to further stretch leg. Do four and alternate with other side for a series. Do four series.

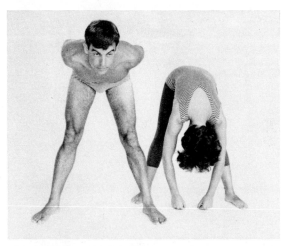

74 FLEXIBILITY BOUNCES Most important of all the flexibility exercises. Stand with feet apart, hands clasped behind back. Lean forward from the hips and KEEP YOUR HEAD UP. Bounce the upper body down in eight short bounces. Then drop both arms downward, loose and relaxed. Let your head and whole upper body hang. Do eight more bounces in this position. BE SURE TO STAY LOOSE AND RELAXED. Alternate with head-up bounces and with head-down bounces for four series. **Exercise should be done as often as possible throughout day.**

WALKING TIPS

- *To walk properly you need good posture (pages 42 and 43), good feet (pages 94 and 95) and good walking habits.*
- *Do you toe in (pigeon toes)? Do exercises **75, 76, 77.***
- *Do you toe out? Do exercise **78.***
- *Do you walk heavily and without spring? Do exercise **79.***
- *Does your walk lack grace? Do exercise **75.***
- *Do your thighs need work? Do exercise **76.***
- *Does your low back tire easily and do you need heel cord stretch? Do exercise **80.***
- *Do you waddle or swing your seat around? Check your leg length. See page 19.*
- *Do these walking exercises to a good brisk rhythm. Leroy Anderson's "Promenade" is good. Then do them to slow rhythms. Do them barefoot and do them often.*

WALKS

75 TURNED-OUT WALK Before you start: head up, chest out, abdominals flat, both shoulders and arms relaxed. Use a crack in the floor, line on a rug or lay a piece of tape. Step forward on line turning right foot out, follow with left foot out. Walk all the way across, then walk the same line back **backwards**. Keep the beat with the feet turned out.

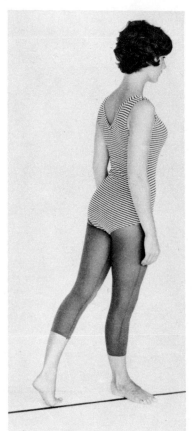

76 TURNED-OUT EXTENDED WALK Take a long step forward with foot turned way out. Try to put toes down first. Go across in forward position and return going **backwards**. Toes must touch first, then heel pressed firmly down and **in**. To futher strengthen thighs, do same extended walk but straighten knees. Go all the way across, then back in half-knee-bent position as if walking under a low roof.

77 CROSSOVER WALK This is an exaggeration of Exercise **75**. Cross right foot **over** line and turn toes way out to point toward it. Then bring left foot around to cross to other side of line with toes pointed sharply out. Go across forward; return walking the same way backward. On the return keep body bent forward as if traveling under same low roof. Reach way back with a turned-out foot.

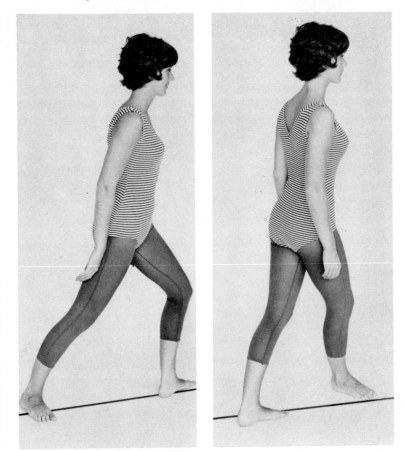

WALKS

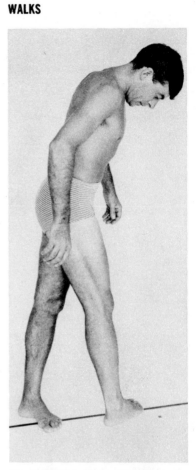

78 TURNED-IN WALK Proceed on line, turning feet in as far as possible with each step. On return, turn around and come back with feet turned in, but with knees slightly bent. This is excellent for muscles on front and outer sides of legs.

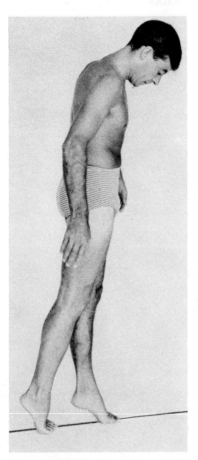

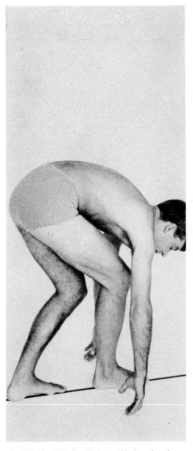

79 TOE BOUNCES Keep knees straight and stiff. Let all the action come from feet. Rise high on toes and walk as close to line as possible with light easy bounces. Return the same way.

80 DROP WALK This will be hard on your back and heel cords. Bend low letting knees bend and fingers drag on floor. Plant heels firmly and keep foot pointed straight ahead, rather than in or out. When you come to the end stand up and walk back naturally to rest your back. Then repeat.

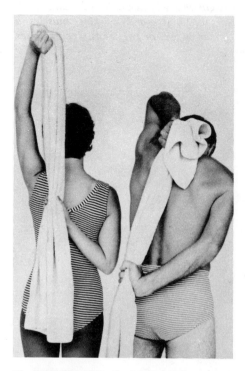

81 SHOULDER PULL Used **isometrically,** towel is held in two hands. Pull one against the other and don't let either win. Hold pull for six seconds and relax. Do two.

ISOMETRIC CONTRACTION TIPS

- *In Isometric Contraction the muscle tenses but does not change in length, and therefore no movement ensues.*
- *When a muscle has contracted to 60% of its potential, circulation stops and no more oxygen reaches the muscle. This is self-limiting.*
- *Isometrics will build strength, but that is virtually all. The body is usually more in need of flexibility, full range of motion in joints and endurance.*

- *Use Isometrics if you wish (exercises* **81** *through* **85***) but know that they are only a small part of an exercise program. If you have a limited time for your program, you would do better to lift weights and build strength this way while at the same time working arm, shoulder and knee joints—and working muscles all along their lengths rather than in one or two spots. See exercises 87–95.*
- *Use Isometrics,* but don't stop there, *three minutes out of any hour's workout is enough for Isometrics.*

82 LEG PRESS Done **isometrically:** Put foot in loop of towel. Pull hard with both hands; at the same time push hard with the foot. Hold for six seconds and release. Alternate feet for two

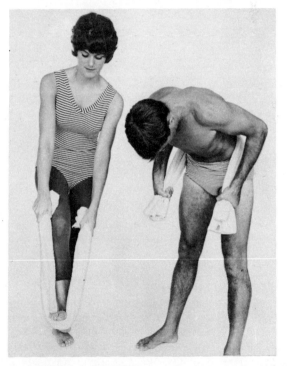

83 ABDOMINAL & ARM PRESS Drape towel over your back, hold the two ends in your hands and push down. Draw in your abdominals hard. Hold the contraction for six seconds. Do two.

84 CHEST STRETCH Grasp ends of towel and stretch it above your head. Try to press it backward over your head to rest on your seat. Don't bend arms. Return back over head the same way keeping tension on towel.

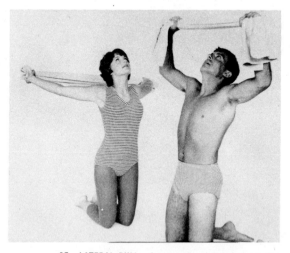

85 LATERAL PULL Grasp ends of towel short. For **isometric** contraction, pull both hands outward simultaneously and hold for six seconds. Do two.

DYNAMIC RESISTANCE TIPS

Far better than pitting one's strength against one's own muscles, a chair, a wall or a machine . . . is work with another human being. To begin with, it's more fun. Secondly, it gives the stronger a sense of strength and responsibility. *When the odds are more even, competition does play a part, but the idea is that of finding the point of balance rather than shoving the other person across the floor.*

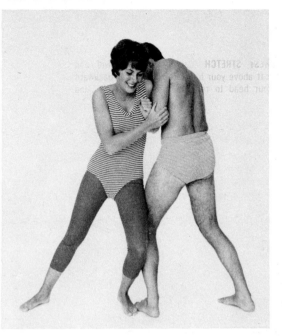

86 PUSH ME—PULL YOU Stand with feet apart, the outsides of the left feet pressed against each other. Place the left arms and shoulders against each other (don't lock arms)—and **push!** Find the balance point (where the weaker partner cannot take any more) and hold that point for ten second. Do the same to the other side.

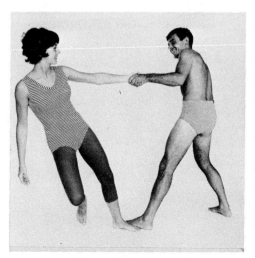

WEIGHT TRAINING TIPS

- *There are several ways to weight train. The safest and best is to work for definition, in which muscles are well defined rather than bulgy and bulky. This is accomplished by lifting lighter weights more often, rather than very heavy weights less often.*
- *Weight training is an excellent strengthener (also for girls—and the muscle strength will not show except as "curves" and in improved function).*
- *Weight bags in graduated weights, one-, two- and five-pounders are very practical, as they are easily stored, will not smash a toe if dropped, and can be used by the whole family.*
- *Weight bags can be hung on a broomstick or just hand-held for the "usual" lifts, and they can be used with all "free" exercises (pages 126–128).*
- *Weight training should be done only every other day and always preceded and followed by warm-up and stretching exercises. On the alternate days running or rope jumping are ideal.*

WEIGHT TRAINING

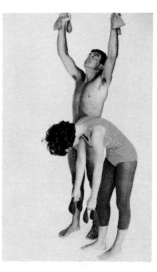

87 OVERHEAD PRESS (Start with light weights and increase as strength grows. Add weight rather than repetitions.) Lean down and touch floor with weights. If weights are light don't bend knees. Raise weights to chest, then press them overhead. Return to chest and back to floor. Do ten **slowly** to slow music (if you are lifting twenty pounds, you will feel it soon enough).

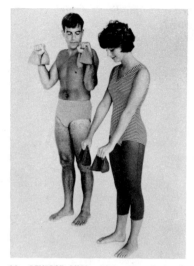

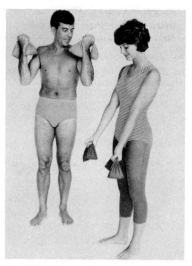

88 REVERSE CURL With palms facing **in**, allow weights to hang at full arm stretch. Then, keeping elbows in, bend arms to bring weights to shoulder level palms facing **out**. Do ten. Alternate with **Exercise 89**, and do twenty of each.

89 CURL Allow weights to hang at full-arm stretch palms facing **out**. Then, with elbows in, bend arms to bring weights to shoulder level, palms facing **in**. Do ten, then alternate with **Exercise 88**, to do twenty of each.

90 KNEE BENDS Place weight on shoulders, or if you want to drape them over a broomstick, place broomstick back of shoulders. Do ten slow deep knee bends.

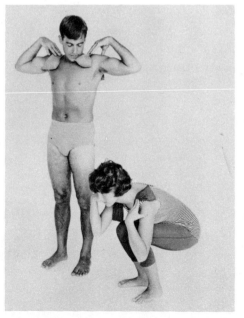

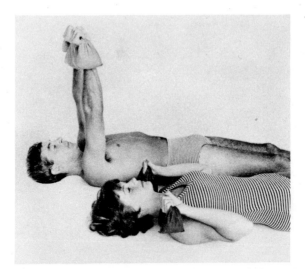

91 BENCH PRESS Lie supine. Extend weights straight up in the air above your face. Bend and stretch for ten and alternate with **Exercise 92**, to do twenty of each.

92 LATERAL EXTENSION Stretch arms straight up so that weights are above your face. With straight arms, lower weights to sides, but do not touch them to floor. (More beneficial if you lie on a piano bench; the chest will be further stretched as the weights pull down below the level of your body—and you have to work harder as they are lifted from that level.) THIS IS **THE** BEST BUST DEVELOPMENT EXERCISE. Do ten and alternate with **Exercise 91** so that you do twenty of each.

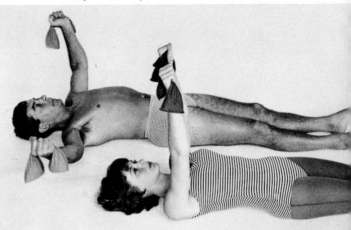

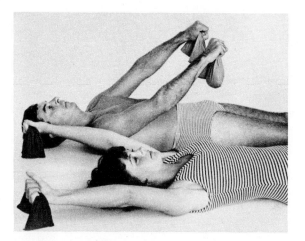

93 OVERHEAD EXTENSION Raise arms straight up in the air. Lower arms over head but do not quite touch the floor. Return to straight-up position and then lower forward but do not quite touch the thighs. Do ten.

To improve, merely add weights. This means you need spend no more time as you continue to overload.

ALWAYS DO FREE EXERCISES AFTER ANY FORM OF WEIGHT TRAINING. (See Page 142).

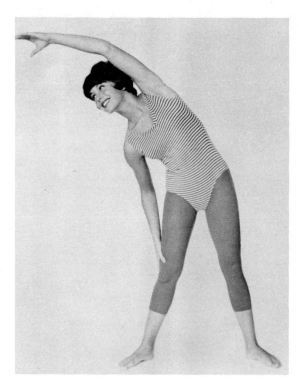

94 OVERARM REACH Stand with feet apart, right hand on right thigh and left hand straight overhead. Slide right hand down thigh to top of your knee and that will draw the left over your head to the right side. In this position bounce down to the side four times. Then swing over to do the same on the other side. That makes a series. Do four series. Carry two or five (or more) pounds in your overhead hand, to increase the efficiency of the exercise.

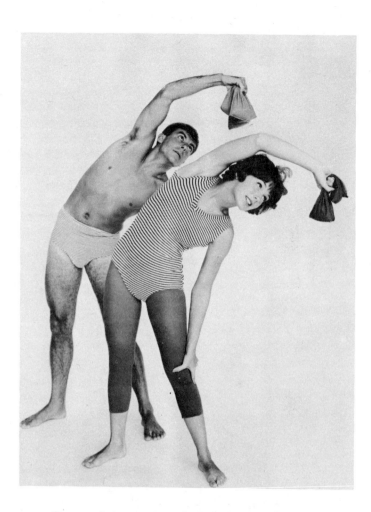

There are three ways to overload muscles and overloading is
what improves strength, endurance and even flexibility. You
can increase repetitions, which takes time. You can speed up,
but that often means that you do your exercises incompletely.
Or you can add weight. This last is the easiest. Almost any
exercise in this book lends itself to weight work.

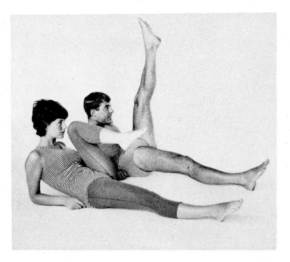

To improve leg strength for any and all sports, merely hang weights on legs. If you lift too high the weights will slide off, of course, but there is no need to lift that high. Adjust your exercise to the equipment.

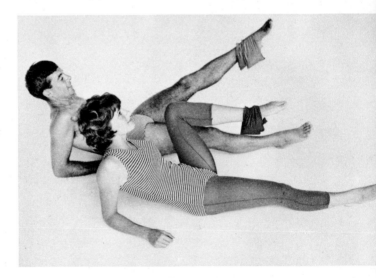

95 LEG EXTENSIONS WITH WEIGHTS Lie supine resting on bent elbows. Draw the weighted left leg in, bending your knee, then extend. Do ten. Change the weights to the other leg and repeat.

RUNNING TIPS

- *To improve endurance, run.*
- *To improve heart action, run.*
- *To improve lung capacity, run.*
- *Running is one of the best exercises. It is a good idea to run over uneven terrain, so that the muscles are being used in constant change as the trail changes in elevation and in surface. If this is not possible, at least change the form of your run. This insures against the same muscles pounding away in the same position with the same intensity, which can, and often does, cause shin splints and muscle strain.*
- *If you have the kind of ankles that turn and knees that ache when you run, check the possibility of the long second toe joint. Put the felt in your sneaks and start easy.*
- *If you haven't run in a long time start easy. Run a few steps in place, say sixteen, then stop. The next day take it up to twenty. If you find you are too breathless drop off a few and build more slowly.*
- *Running to music is the best way to keep up a steady beat and enjoy it.*
- *Do exercises* **96–101.**

RUNNING

96 RUNNING IN PLACE Using a good fast record to keep you going in time (Leroy Anderson's "Fiddle Faddle" is great) run for sixteen steps. Land on your toes but bring foot down on heel at each step—keep it light.

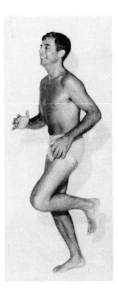

WARNING:

NEVER RUN BEFORE MUSCLES ARE WARM
(See Page 142)

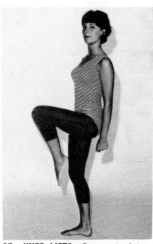

97 KNEE LIFTS For next sixteen steps, lift knees high and point toes to stretch insteps.

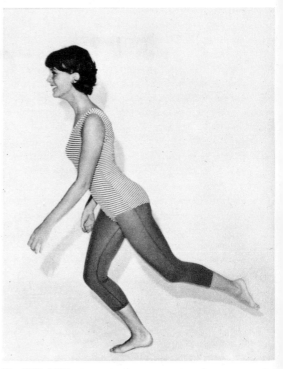

98 KICK BACK On next sixteen steps lean forward swinging arms freely and kicking your legs out behind.

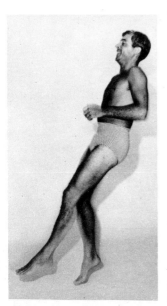

99 KICK FORWARD Finally, lean back and bring straight legs forward for sixteen. Repeat the series.

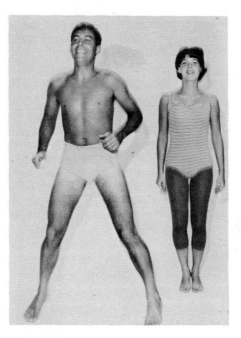

100 APART-TOGETHER Jumping the feet apart and together works the legs two different ways. Do sixteen. DO NOT CLAP HANDS OVER HEAD.

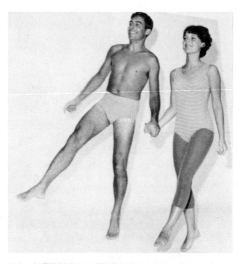

101 ALTERNATING HOPS Hop eight times on the left foot and then eight on the right to make up a series. Do four.

JUMP ROPE TIPS

- *Jumping rope is one of the quickest and best ways to condition your heart.*
- *Take your pulse before jumping, jump for one minute at one jump per second and take your pulse again. Rest for one minute and take it again. Take it once more five minutes later. Check with the heart section on page 20 to see what this can mean to you.*
- *Out of doors try to progress by combining running with rope jumping.*
- *Rope jumping can be used as good interval training: jump lazily for sixteen jumps, then as fast as you can for eight, lazily for another sixteen and fast for eight. That would be a series; start with one and slowly build as endurance improves.*

JUMP ROPE. If you have never jumped rope: stand feet together, loop of rope in back of you. Swing rope over your head by using hands and wrists, **not the whole arm.** When loop is in front, step over it. Repeat and when you can anticipate falling loop, try to jump over it **once.** Repeat several times, then try for two jumps without stopping. Gradually increase.

102 DOUBLE LEG JUMPS. Jump with both feet at same time. At first you will jump once for every swing of the rope. To take it easy at first, slow rope to point where you jump over it on one count and jump a second smaller jump while it is directly overhead. Speed up by jumping once each time rope comes around. Double the rope's speed.

103 ALTERNATING LEG JUMPS You can alternate legs and jump over the rope every time it comes around, or you can slow the rope so that you hop twice on one foot for each swing.

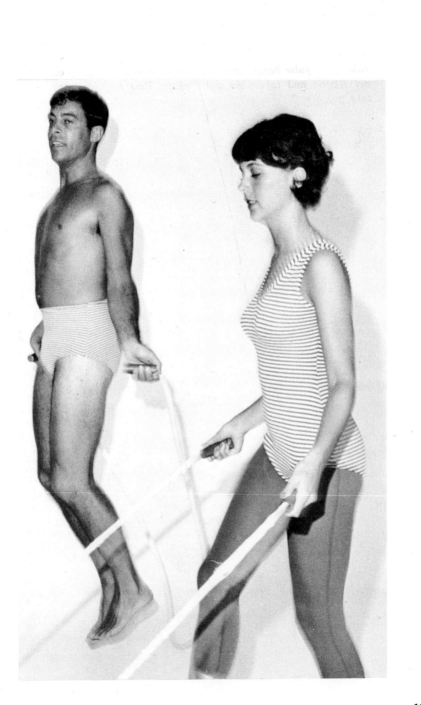

PRE AND POST NATAL EXERCISE TIPS

- *Having a baby can be a wonderful experience if you are in shape for it. That means having strong flexible muscles, the ability to relax at will, and normal weight.*
- *About 50% of America's women are not in that condition, so they put on even more weight which is hard to lose later on. They have backaches, their feet and legs hurt, they are hungry and tired all the time. All unnecessary!*
- *Your baby needs a good hotel to grow in. That means you must be active to keep your circulation good and burn up calories so that you need not starve to keep your weight down. You must use and strengthen the muscles you will need in the delivery room, flexible muscles that relax when you tell them to.*
- *Do your exercises for nine months before the baby . . . and start working at regaining your figure right after the baby.*
- *Do exercises **104–112**.*

PRE- AND POST-NATAL EXERCISES

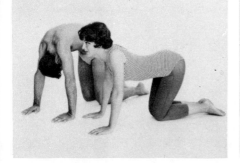 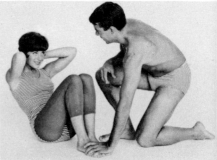

104 CAT & OLD HORSE Start on hands and knees. Drop head and look at your abdomen. Let it go slack. Then tighten the abdominal muscles and pull in. Holding them tight, arch your back up into the angry cat position and hold for three counts. Next, drop your back down into the sag of an old swaybacked horse. Alternate for four.

105 ROLL-DOWNS & SIT-UPS If when you took the tests on page 61 you passed test #2, just keep right on doing those sit-ups—five of them four times a day. If you couldn't pass the test, then start with ROLL-DOWNS (Exercise 2). Try to get those abdominals in shape and keep them that way.

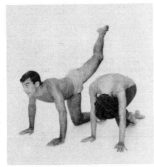

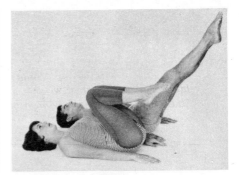

106   KNEE - TO - NOSE KICK
Pregnant women often develop a flabby seat. This causes backache and is hard to get rid of later. Keep your gluteals firm; you will need them at delivery. Kneeling, bring knee as close to nose as possible. As you begin to bulge bring knee forward a little to the side. Do four on each side for a series. Do two and alternate with **Exercise 107** to do four series of each.

107 SPINE-DOWN STRETCH This helps your abdominals and also prevents tendancy to swayback. Lie supine, knees bent, spine pressed tight to floor. Extend straight legs overhead, then return to rest. On the second extension, lower legs just a few inches but be sure your spine is still flat on the floor. Bring knees in to "rest." Keep extending and drawing until you no longer can keep spine down flat. At that point you have gone too low . . . go back to the last spine-flat extension and do five. Alternate with **Exercise 106**, so that you do two series of each.

IF AT ANY TIME YOU FEEL ANY BACK DISCOMFORT, GET DOWN ON THE FLOOR AND DO THE LIMBERING SERIES, EXERCISES 12a, b, c, d, e.

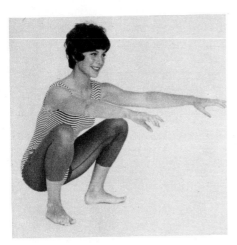

108 OPEN KNEE BEND You will need strong legs as you grow heavier—and you don't want to get fat pneumatic thighs—so do knee bends. The open knee bend will help with crotch flexibility, but add **Exercises 71, 72** and **67** to make sure you have it.

PRE- AND POST-NATAL RELAXATION

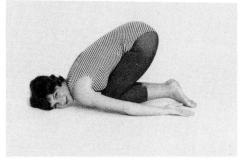

109 KNEE CHEST REST To relieve pressure from the growing child inside you, kneel on slightly spread knees. Put one ear on floor and bring both arms to rest on floor alongside legs. Rest for one minute like this, then change head so that other ear rests on floor. Two minutes gives you back some stretch and rests your pelvic area.

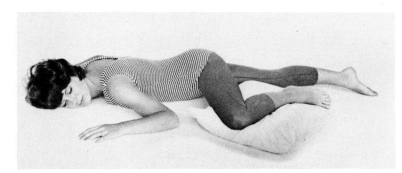

110 PRONE REST, ONE PILLOW A tired back rests best with one knee bent whether you are prone or supine. The pillow under the knee changes the angle of the pelvis and takes further strain off of the back. It also makes room for expanding tummy.

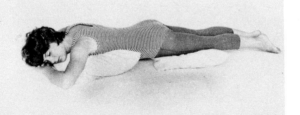

111 PRONE REST, TWO PILLOWS For those who have rested prone all their lives, the sudden appearance of a bulge in front can be distressing. If you want to lie face down, put a pillow above and below your bulge, and go ahead.

IF FATHERS-TO-BE WILL DO THESE EXERCISES TOO . . . BOTH WILL HAVE SLENDER, STRONG FIGURES AFTER D-DAY!

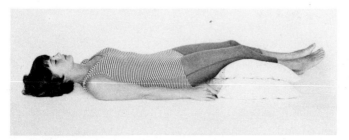

112 SUPINE REST When you rest on your back, put a pillow under your knees. The elevated position will help your legs. Circulation is often slowed because of the weight of the child against the large veins coming up into the pelvis. With elevated legs, circulation will increase which will make you less tired, your feet and ankles less swollen, and help to prevent varicose veins.

RELAXATION TIPS

- *Because there is so much unrelieved stress in our lives, we find true relaxation hard to come by.*
- *Just saying, "Now I'm going to relax," rarely brings either relaxation or sleep.*

RELAXATION

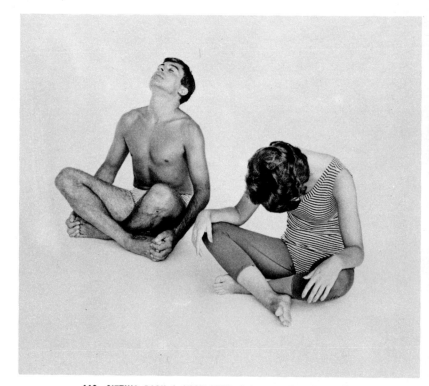

113 SITTING BACK & NECK REST Cats can relax, they make a business of it. Humans can relax too **if the pressure is off.**

- Relaxation comes best *after* a thorough physical workout.
- *Children, in particular, need (and do not get) tremendous doses of activity if they are to sleep early and well.*
- *The more stress in any given day, the more you will need to physically work it off, before you can relax.*

You can't do it before the pressure is off because it is also human nature to be ready for the worst. If you have just been through an unpleasant experience, a quarrel, a sorrow, a loss or a crisis, don't just suffer and grow tight and miserable.

Do something very active like a long, **fast** walk.

Exercise until the sweat pours off you.

Run.

Then take a shower and sit down alone, all alone. Let your head fall forward and hang. Concentrate on the hanging. Concentrate on the pull as it works down the spine where all your tense and jangling nerves are waiting. Rest your arms and let your hands hang. Then turn your concentration from the pulling back to the hanging hands . . . back and forth. Let go everywhere you can find a tense spot.

From time to time sit up, take a huge breath and lean your head back just for a moment . . . then repeat the hang. After five minutes you will feel no happier, no less angry, nothing will have changed except one thing. You will be able to handle it without damage to yourself.

Watch people as they fidget through life, scratching, picking, biting nails, wringing their hands. **DON'T.** Cultivate relaxation as you would practice the piano or your golf stroke. You will be less tired, less tense, and much nicer to be with.

RELAXATION AFTER EXERCISE—AND BEFORE SLEEP

FOR MANY PEOPLE PLEASANT SOFT MUSIC IS AN AID TO RELAX-
ATION. AFTER YOU HAVE DONE YOUR EXERCISES—AND YOU
SHOULD END THEM WITH SOMETHING STRENUOUS LIKE THE
RUNNING EXERCISES OR ROPE JUMPING TAPERING OFF WITH
THREE OR FOUR MINUTES OF "WARM-UPS" (PAGE **142**)—LIE
DOWN AND "TALK" YOURSELF THROUGH THIS RELAXATION
EXERCISE.

114 SUPINE & SIDE REST Start supine; many people find that
bending one knee rests their backs. Close your eyes and talk
it down—hypnotically:
INHALE VERY SLOWLY
EXHALE
INHALE
EXHALE
YOUR HEAD IS RESTING
AND YOUR NECK
LET GO IN YOUR SHOULDERS
YOUR UPPER ARMS
LET GO IN YOUR ELBOWS
YOUR LOWER ARMS
WRISTS
FINGERS
INHALE VERY DEEPLY
EXHALE
INHALE SLOWLY
EXHALE
SHOULDERS ARE RESTING
RELAX YOUR BACK
YOUR WAIST IS RESTING
YOUR HIPS
LET GO IN YOUR THIGHS
YOUR KNEES
THE BACK OF YOUR LEGS
ANKLES
HEELS
INSTEPS
TOES
INHALE . . . EXHALE . . .
INHALE . . . EXHALE
Then go back and do the whole thing again saying it slower and
slower, taking deeper and deeper breaths. Try to find every
tense tight spot and **let go.** Roll over on one side and repeat.

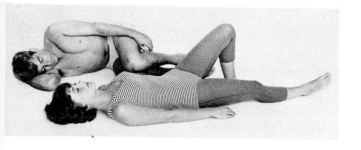

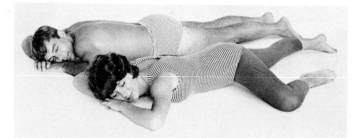

115 PRONE REST Lie prone and try the "talk-down" if you prefer that position, but when you do lie prone try bringing one or the other leg out to the side where it can rest your lower back. If you are given to low back trouble at all, it would be well to do the limbering exercises 12a, b, c, d, e, and **19 before** you start your "talk-down".

WARM-UP EXERCISES

- *Warm-ups are designed to actually warm your muscles (a warm muscle is 20% more efficient than a cold one, and therefore less prone to injury). They loosen stiff joints, increase circulation and take nothing out of you.*
- *Warm-ups should be used before any sport or spike activity. Many ski accidents, as well as tennis elbows, pitcher's arms and even football knees, would be avoided if proper warm-ups were used each time before the sport is begun.*
- *Ideal warm-up exercises:* **23, 31, 36, 27, 43, 22, 61,** *and* **74,** *in that order.*
- *Never spend more than 15 seconds on any one exercise, but move on to a different area. The above program starts with "swims" to relax shoulders; 31 is a waist worker; 36 goes for hips and thighs; 27 for arms and chest; 43 for thighs and crotch; 22 for shoulders and arms again; 61 for knees and feet; 29 for quick warming; and finally, 74 for flexibility.*
- *To cool off after your heavy program use exercises 23, 31 and 32.*

THE EXERCISE PROGRAM

- *Everyone needs exercise but not always the same exercises and not to the same degree. Check with your problems through the tests (pages 11–16) the measurements (pages 17–19) and with posture (page 41). Know which five exercises you are going to start with.*
- *When you do your exercises doesn't matter.*
- *Wear comfortable clothes that don't bind.*
- *Exercises in this book will not tire you. They will stimulate you. Instead of taking a pep pill before you go to the party, do ten minutes of exercise, take a shower, and feel the difference—you will glow!*
- *Music is an invaluable aid. Use it whenever you can.*
- *Start with warm-ups. Go on to strength exercises, then flexibility. Wind up with runs and a few more warm-ups which will cool you down.*
- *Start with ten minutes a day—and whatever else you do, do those exercises regularly.*

HOW TO CONDUCT A CLASS IN PHYSICAL EDUCATION

- *There is a demand for exercises to be given in conjunction with sports programs. This book can provide many shortcuts.*
- *Start with the minimum test on page 12. It takes 90 seconds per child and locates main weaknesses which must be repaired before heavy exercise or sports can be undertaken.*
- *Follow with optimum test (page 15) or any other optimum test, provided it includes flexibility.*
- *Next check the information on establishing an exercise program (page 143).*
- *Place the class in a circle, put on a record with a brisk popular tune.*
- *Start with the warm-up exercises on page 146 and be sure to change often. But never do any one exercise for more than fifteen or twenty seconds.*
- *From warm-ups go to sitting floor exercises:* **35, 41, 44, 45, 46, 67.** *Vary the music, either fast or slow. Do the exercises to the music. Slowly is more difficult.*
- *From sitting exercises, roll back to the supine position and do exercises* **17** *and* **35.**
- *Next go to kneeling exercises:* **16, 19, 33, 37, 38.**
- *Finish off with runs (on pages 129–133). And relaxation (page 138).*
- *If you have only 10 minutes, start with warm-ups and use one or two from each of the other groups.*
- *For people with posture problems check with posture section.*
- *For specific exercises for pre-sport programs check with pre-sport exercises on page 145.*
- *Girls are primarily interested in their figures. These are the specific exercises they will need:*
- *Abdominals, exercise* **2** • *Thighs, exercise* **41** • *Waist, exercise* **31**
- *Bust, exercises* **27** *and* **92.** • *Hips, exercises* **37** *and* **38** • *Fibrositis, pages 27, 101, 102.*
- *Boys are over-tight and over-tense. They will need flexibility exercises* after warm-ups. *Give them exercises:* **74, 26, 27, 30, 56, 67, 68, 69, 71, 72, 73.**
- *If exercises are to be taught in the classrooms, use all standing exercises starting with warm-ups and ending with runs.*

PRE-SPORT TRAINING

- *You get in shape to ski, you don't ski to get in shape. And that goes for all other sports. Reverse the process and the least you will get is sore muscles; if you ski, you may break a leg.*
- *Get in shape for sport with exercises, but warm up for exercises with warm-ups (see page 142).*
- *The following exercises are specifics for each sport:*
  baseball, football, basketball, soccer, tennis, handball, squash—3, 10, 14, 15, 17, 23, 26, 29, 33, 56, 57, 58 and pages 110–113 and 129–133.
  Golf—3, 4, 13, 17, 21, 31, 32, 57, 58.
  Swimming—4, 7, 10, 11, 13, 14, 15, 17, 18, 19, 21, 22, 23, 26, 28, 30, 33, 35, 37, 39, 46, 50, 56, 59, 61 and pages 110–113 and 129–133.
  Gymnastics, the dance, figure skating, cheerleading—3, 7, 8, 11, 13, 14, 15, 18, 19, 22, 26, 28, 29, 30, 32, 33, 36, 39, 43, 44, 45, 62a, 62b, and pages 110–113 and 129–133.
  Riding—5, 6, 7, 8, 10, 14, 23, 26, 27, 36, 37, 38.
  Skiing—8, 11, 14, 15, 17, 29, 30, 43, 56, 61, 71, 72, 74, and pages 80–83 and 129–133.
  Boxing, wrestling, fencing—3, 4, 8, 11, 14, 15, 21, 22, 25, 27, 28, 34, 35, 36, 38, 43, 45, 50, 51, 52, 58, 59, 60, 61, 74, 76 and pages 110–113 and 129–133.
- *Anyone going out for any sport should do weight training (pages 122–125).*
- *Anyone going out for any sport should realize that flexibility will probably be the deciding factor, and prepare for it. Once you are actually working in the sport, strength is going to improve but flexibility may not. If there is tension produced by your sport you will become even less flexible. So work for flexibility in your daily workouts.*
- *If you don't have time for all the exercises, note where you left off and continue from that point at your next session.*

OCCUPATIONAL HAZARDS (*EVERY* OCCUPATION HAS THEM)

To ward off occupational muscle pain:

Workers who sit, do exercises 32, 36, 37;

   Who tighten legs around chair legs, do exercises 43, 45, 46;
   Who hunch over at their work, do exercises 26, 27;
   Who relax abdominals continuously, do exercises 2, 8, 17;
   Who build up tension in thighs, do exercises 41, 43;
   Who build up tension in neck and shoulders, do exercises 20, 21, 22, 23.

Houseworkers who stand still a lot at tasks, do exercises 59, 60, 61;

   Who lift heavy objects, do exercises 12, 13, 16;
   Who tighten up in neck and shoulders, do exercises 20, 21, 23.

Stand-up workers like shopkeepers, dentists, surgeons, assembly liners, do exercises 50, 51, 52, 56, 59, 60, 61, 62;

   Who often work in awkward positions, do exercises 23, 27;
   Who tighten shoulders and back muscles, do exercises 12, 20, 21;
   Who breathe poorly and have poor circulation, do exercises 102, 103;
   Who develop varicose veins, see page 74.

Drivers—Car, bus (train, plane)—who develop tension from the concentration called for in staying alive on today's highways, do exercises 22, 23, 115;

   Who develop low back pain, do exercises 9, 12, 16;
   Who have poor circulation, do exercises 50, 52, 71, 72, 74;
   Who develop hemorrhoids, see page 23;
   Who get tension headaches often, do exercises 20, 21, 64a, 64b;
   Who develop bursitis, do exercises 24, 25.

Heavy workers build strength but often lack flexibility, which means they not only fight the job, but much of the time work against their own strength when muscles don't relax properly. Their prime need is increased muscle flexibility, acquired by doing exercises 4, 8, 12, 20, 21, 23, 27, 31, 56; and the exercises on pages 110–113, 138–141 for relaxation.

PHYSICAL FITNESS AND INDUSTRY

- *Millions of man and woman hours are lost yearly because both executives and employees are physically unfit. They are tired, lack resistance to disease, lack stamina, enthusiasm and drive. They are prey to emotional disorders, the women to menstrual disorders, and many young men die of heart attacks at the peak of their careers.*
- *If industry wants to cut its personnel loss, improve efficiency and raise production, it must institute physical fitness for both executives and employees—on company time and at company expense. The hook? If you don't stay fit, you don't work here.*
- *Needed for executive fitness: A room 20 x 40 feet; weight bags, jump ropes, record player; an exercise teacher; showers (or sauna); at least two sessions a week, one half hour each.*
- *Needed for employee fitness: A large room (cafeteria) that can be used after hours; jump ropes, balance beams, weight bags, record player; showers and an exercise teacher; at least one one-hour session each week.*
- *Those industries that employ people to work long hours at tables should offer a five-minute exercise session, doing exercises* **20, 21, 22, 23, 26, 27, 31, 32, 36, 43, 50, 59, 61, 96,** *morning and afternoon. This would lessen fatigue, cut down obesity, improve emotional health and increase both production and product quality.*
- *When industry knows that people make just as much difference to production as machines, there will be a vast improvement in national health.*

HANDICAPS

- *No matter what your physical handicap, there is always* something *to be done. First ask yourself what has been affected, then what is left to you, and finally what you must augment to help compensate for handicap areas.*
- *Blindness: You can't see, but the rest of your body can be worked, reflexes made faster, strength and flexibility improved and emotional stress relieved. You need abdominal strength (pages 25 through 30); back stretch and strength (pages 35 through 40) to support all the rest. Add flexibility (pages 110 through 113) and foot exercises for balance (pages 94 through 98). And you will need stamina (pages 118 through 131). With the body you can build, you can go anywhere.*
- *Deafness calls for the same program, plus pages 48 through 59.*
- *Brain damaged people need rhythm, and simple patterning. Have them do exercises 4,* **9, 12,** *16,* **20, 21, 22, 23,** *27,* **29, 31, 33, 37, 41,** *and pages 114–117, 131–137.*

BED PATIENT OR WHEELCHAIR PATIENT

- *Bed patient or wheelchair patient: see the chair exercises pages 100 through 103.*
- *Amputation: whatever limb was lost, you will need much trunk work to strengthen the stabilizing area. Do exercises* **5, 6, 7, 8, 9, 10, 11, 12.**
- *Post-operative: anyone who has had an operation will be handicapped for a little while, but most operations are to help you get back into life, not give you an excuse to stay out. The incision will heal, and no, it won't come apart the first time you bend over. Start with the chair exercises on pages 100 through 103. Progress to the limbering series pages 35 through 37. Continue on with warm-ups (see page 142), and you are on your way.*
- *Mastectomy: should mean nothing except that you had an operation. Do as the other post-ops do and add exercises* **21, 22, 23, 24, 25, 26, 27, 31, 32, 33.**
- *Arthritis: there are several kinds. If your doctor says exercise, look up the affected area in the table of contents and begin.*

CHRONIC PROBLEMS

- *The word "chronic" means lasting a long time, but that doesn't mean "ruin your life." Physical fitness can do a lot to make life easier and even lessen the chronic problem in many cases.*
- *Diabetes: exercise is known to lessen the need for insulin.*
- *Multiple sclerosis: a disease that has a pattern of "mountains" when you feel well and "valleys" when you are having an attack. It is important to make use of the "mountains" to get your body in the best possible shape so that the "valleys" will not bring you so low. Full range of motion for all joints, and considerable attention to flexibility, as well as trunk strength.*
- *Hypertension: also helped with exercise. If you have given up activity because you can't go in for the violent sports you used to like, take up exercise. Feel better, get better . . . and who knows?*
- *Poor balance: if your balance is impaired you are afraid to take the chance of falling when being active. Result is your muscles are deteriorating and inflexibility is making you old. You can do most exercises in this book on the floor or holding on to someone. Make yourself strong and flexible so that when you do lose your balance you don't fall on your face.*
- *Chronic Backache: (see backs on pages 31 through 34). There are very few bad backs that being stronger, more flexible and emotionally relaxed won't help (see also page 151 on emotional stress).*

EMOTIONAL STRESS

- *Your body and your emotions are interrelated. If one is in trouble, the other becomes involved.*
- *The human body needs physical outlet for stress; the more stress the more outlet needed. If either the opportunity or the vehicle (a good body) is missing, the body will take it out on itself. Then we see tension headaches, the tension syndrome, stiff and painful shoulders, upper and low back pain, muscle cramps in legs, menstrual cramps, ulcers, and a host of other unpleasantnesses.*
- *When you are under very great stress and can take time out for a long hike through the country, a noon swim and a rub down, a game of tennis or golf, a dance or an exercise class, you get rid of some of the pressure on you. Just try it! Physical outlets are a must if you are to remain on an even keel.*
- *If you find you are drinking too much, you need the physical outlet to relax your tensions (the ones you are trying to wet down) and you need to break out of the pattern of being where the drinks and the drinking companions are.*
- *If your business is in trouble, you need the physical outlets that will cut the problems down to size when you feel relaxed and rested.*
- *If retirement is looming and it worries you, you need physical outlets to relieve the stress and also to build you up to face and take on a different life.*
- *Teenagers need physical outlets in order to lessen their special emotional tensions, keep sexual needs at a level where they don't constantly intrude, and to give them a self-image that pleases them.*

AGING

- *With proper diet and exercise the aging process can be slowed considerably. If you have "let yourself go," you can reverse the process.*
- *Very few fat people live to be old (see section on obesity, page 153).*
- *Is your gait old? That isn't age, it is disuse. (See feet and legs, pages 94, 96, 74.)*
- *Do your knees or hips give you trouble? (See pages 78, 68 and 72.) Incidentally, those exercises to reduce hips and thighs will also oil the joints.*
- *Does your back bother you? (See page 34.)*
- *Stiff shoulders? (See page 51.)*
- *Stiff knees? Walking around on legs that hurt doesn't make sense. Do the exercises that will strengthen and relax them and improve your circulation. (See knees, page 77; foot massage, page 96; and a few simple exercises that will help: 40, 41, 42, 44, 45, 46). And whenever you can, get your feet higher than your head.*
- *The chair exercises on pages 100 through 103 can be done any time.*
- *When no one is around who might think you had taken leave of your senses, turn on a record or the radio and do the walks across the room (pages 114 through 117).*
- *Always keep in mind that if you built a body before you were twelve, it is still there waiting to be reclaimed.*

OBESITY

- *Almost no obesity is "Glandular."*
- *A great deal of obesity, even in children, is caused by emotional disturbance.*
- *Obesity is often due not just to how much we eat, but what we eat.*
- *Obesity is not hereditary—but family eating habits have a lot to do with making children look like their obese parents. If two parents are fat the children have an 80% chance of being fat.*
- *Obesity is a contributing factor to many diseases.*
- *No one who is obese can be physically attractive, no matter how pleasant they try to be.*
- *Calories do count, so count them, but remember you need some food so make what you eat count.*
- *Many foods contain "empty calories," calories that count toward making you fat but do not provide the nutrition you need.*
- *Exercise does count in obesity and it can help take weight off.*
- *If you combine exercise with diet, weight comes off and muscles tone (to take up slack).*
- *When you start on your particular program, weight should be noted every day. If it goes down, be pleased. If it goes up, go light on food that day. Don't wait for the end of the year, the end of the month or even the end of the week to find out what is going on in you. And be aware that the slow, sneaky two or three pounds a year are the hardest to get off.*

DIET

There is even more confusion about diet than there has been about exercise, mostly because both have been discussed so loudly by people who really know nothing about either. Here are some facts you should know:

- Fat by any other name is still fat and Americans consume too much of it. It has proven that in countries with a low fat diet people are thinner and have far fewer heart attacks than Americans who average much fatter with a disastrous heart attack rate.

- The body requires energy from food to function. The heavier the job, the more energy needed, and therefore the more food. But conversely, the less active the job, the less energy needed, and therefore less food.

- While all foods contain calories, not all foods provide much energy. That's why you feel you must eat and eat and eat again. Notable among the foods that provide only "empty calories" are those that have been denatured by commercial food manufacturers such as sugar, highly refined flour and saturated fats. The worst are foods that combine all three, such as most commercial baked goods.

- You should not only know which foods are "empty" but you should make a study of the caloric values of all foods. Suppose you are going to have a cocktail before dinner. You might want a Manhattan, but that cocktail has 200 calories. A Martini has 125, Scotch 115 and gin 85. You can add. Two Manhattans will be 400, but two scotches are only a little more than one Manhattan. If you loathe everything but Manhattans and you know one leads to three, have tomato juice: 21 calories.

- With your cocktail you may have to make a choice between 4 ounces of almonds at 425 or peanuts at 670. Cheese may be served; Cheddar is 115, while Munster is 55. Soups differ too, you can have cream of asparagus at 200 or beef bouillon at 10. There are any number in between.

- When it comes to the main course, there are short ribs at 485 or sirloin at 250, but leg of lamb at 230 is less than half the first mentioned. If you prefer fish there is fish stew at 600 or baked sole at 80.

- Vegetables are as controversial. An avocado will cost you 350 calories, potatoes and limas 100, but you can have cauliflower, cabbage or cucumbers for 15.

- When it comes to dessert choose between chocolate ice cream at 400 or flavored gelatin at 75. "What!" you moan, "give up everything I love?" Certainly not, but make those things special, not everyday. If your scale and measurements say you are losing weight nicely, then splurge occasionally. *But if it has another tale to tell and your belt feels snug, settle for a couple of austere weeks.*

- *Even the food processors present choices. Some Maple syrups have labels saying "PURE MAPLE SYRUP" but only 9% of the concoction in the can or bottle is* maple *syrup (though pure). The rest is sugar and corn syrup. You'd be better off buying* pure *100% honey at a Health Food Store. READ THE LABELS ON THE FOODS YOU BUY. . . . A GOODLY PROPORTION IS NUTRITIONALLY WORTHLESS. Choose wisely.*

- *Lastly, you can choose the way in which your food is prepared. Broiled is better than fried. Less cooking is better than too much. Raw fruits and vegetables will help with your vitamin supply. Cover cooking food rather than let it lose considerable value through oxidation. Keep the heat lower than higher. Choose nutrition over appearance and leave the skins on when you can. Potatoes* in the skin *are a great source of potassium . . . you'll be tired if you lack it.*

- *See page 156 for a list of foods with their caloric value. Go over them carefully and cross out the ones you feel you ought to give up because the calories cost is too high. Put a star next to the "safe" ones you can use often, either because you like them or because their low caloric value will give you a chance to indulge somewhere else. In this land of plenty, all you have to do is make the right choices.*

CALORIC VALUE OF FOODS

Per 4 Ounces (Except
Where Otherwise Indicated)

A

Alcohol (per ounce, 90 proof)	360
Alexander cocktail (2 ounces)	225
Almonds (dried)	425
Anchovies (6)	65
Anchovies (1 tablespoon of paste)	40
Anchovies (salted)	160
Apple (medium size)	60
Apple (baked and sugared)	200
Apple juice (1 small glass)	60
Apple pie (1 slice)	350
Apricots (canned—4 halves)	100
Apricots (fresh—three medium)	60
Apricot juice (1 small glass)	75
Artichoke (large)	75
Asparagus (canned)	25
Asparagus (fresh)	25
Avocado (1 small)	350

B

Bacon (grilled—2 small slices)	115
Banana	100
Banana cream pie (1 slice)	260
Beans (green)	20
Beans (canned green)	20
Beans (yellow)	15
Beef:	
boiled beef	240
bouillon cube (1)	3
corned beef	275
hamburger (lean)	245
heart	180
roast beef, T-bone steak, fillet	295
roasted ribs	350
rump	420
short ribs	485
shoulder	180
sirloin	250
smoked beef	300
tail	130
tongue	270
Beer (8 oz.)	130
Beets (red)	35
Benedictine (2 oz.)	160
Baking powder biscuits (2)	260
Blood sausage	480
Brains	120
Brazil nuts (2)	95
Bread (rye slice)	60
Bread (white) slice	65
Bread (whole wheat) slice	55
Brussels Sprouts	60
Butter (salt or sweet—1 oz.)	200
Buttermilk (8 oz.)	85

C

Cabbage (green—raw)	15
Cabbage (red—cooked)	20
Cake (chocolate layer—1 piece)	350
Cake (sponge—1 piece)	120
Canapes (1 small)	30 to 50
Cantaloupe (½)	30
Capers (1 tablespoon)	10
Caramel (1 candy)	45
Carrots (raw—medium)	20
Cauliflower	15
Caviar (1 oz.)	70
Celery (2 stalks)	10
Champagne (1 cup)	90 to 120
Cheese: (per oz.)	
Blue	100
Brie	100
Camembert	85
Cheddar	115
Cottage	25
Cream	105
Gouda	90
Gorgonzola	100
Grated cheese	60
Head	90
Longhorn	90
Munster	55
Neufchatel	100
Parmesan	110
Provolone	95

Roquefort	105
Swiss	105
Cherries (canned)	60
Cherries (fresh)	65
Cherry liqueur (2 oz.)	200
Cherry pie (1 slice)	340
Chestnuts (fresh)	200
Chicory (5 or 6 leaves)	20
Chili Sauce (1 tablespoon)	25
Chives (chopped—1 tablespoon)	1
Chocolate sauce—1 tablespoon	65
Chocolate (milk chocolate)	600
Chocolate meringue pie (1 slice)	275
Cider	50
Clams (12)	100
Coca Cola (8 oz.)	105
Coconut meat (fresh)	165
Codfish (fresh)	80
Codfish (dried)	400
Coffee (black)	0
Cognac (1 oz.)	86
Conger Eel	180
Corn on the cob (1 ear)	85
Crabmeat	120
Crackers (4)	60
Crème de Cacao (1 oz.)	85
Crème de Menthe (1 oz.)	85
Cream (heavy—1 tablespoon)	50
Cream (light—1 tablespoon)	30
Cream (whipped—1 tablespoon)	50
Cream (sour—½ cup)	245
Crepes	230
Crisco	900
Cucumber	15
Currants (fresh—1 cup)	60

D

Daiquiri (1 cocktail)	125
Dandelion greens (1 cup cooked)	80
Dates	300
Dates (Stuffed)	160
Duck (roast)	290 to 360

E

Eclair	300
Eel (fresh)	210
Eel (smoked)	350
Eggplant	30

Endives	25
Endive with butter (1 portion)	100

Eggs:

Egg white	15
Egg yolk	60
Egg (whole)	75
Duck egg	125
Fish eggs (5 oz.)	185
Goose egg	125
Hard boiled egg (1)	75
Omelette (with 1 egg)	105
Poached egg (1)	75
Scrambled egg (1)	105
Soft boiled egg (1)	75
Turkey egg	135

F

Farina cooked—1 cup	105
Figs (canned—3)	125
Figs (dried)	280
Figs (fresh—3 small)	90
Flounder	80
Flour (buckwheat—8 oz.)	340
Flour (rye—8 oz.)	285
Flour (soybean—8 oz.)	230
Flour (wheat—8 oz.)	400
Foie gras (liver paste)	800
Frog legs	85

G

Galantine (pork, veal or fowl)	240
Garlic (clove)	5
Gelatine dessert (plain)	75
Gin (1 oz.)	85
Gin Collins (1 cocktail)	200
Gin Fizz (1 cocktail)	200
Gin Ricky (1 cocktail)	200
Goose (roast)	290 to 360
Grapefruit (½)	75
Grapefruit juice	65
Grapes	50
Gravy (without flour— 1 tablespoon)	100

H

Haddock (1 small portion)	150
Ham (fatty)	440
Ham (grilled)	250
Ham (lean)	145

Hazelnuts	600	Marshmellow (1)	25
Herring (Atlantic)	220	Martini (1 cocktail)	125
Herring (Pacific)	100	Mayonnaise (1 tablespoon)	100
Herring (Kippered)	240	Meringue pie (1 slice)	350
Herring and sour cream	245	Milk (evaporated, unsweetened)	135
Hollandaise Sauce		Milk (condensed, sweetened)	360
(1 tablespoon)	45	Milk (goat's)	85
Honey (1 tablespoon)	60	Milk (skimmed—8 oz.)	85
Honeydew melon (1 slice)	55	Milk (sour)	70
Horse-radish (grated—1 tbs.)	5	Milk (whole—8 oz.)	165
Horse-radish sauce (1 tbs.)	10	Muffin, English (1)	150
Hot dog (1)	100 to 150	Mullet	80
		Mushrooms	15
I		Mussels	95
Ice Cream (chocolate—1 portion)	400	Mustard (1 tablespoon)	10
Ice cream soda	350	Mutton:	
Ice cream sundae	400	Leg of mutton	230
		Mutton chop	350
J		Mutton kidney (broiled)	130
Jams (1 tablespoon)	55	Mutton stew	275
Jellies (fruit jelly—1 tablespoon)	50	Ribs	350
		Shoulder	250
K			
Ketchup (1 tablespoon)	20	**N**	
		Nectarines (2 medium)	60
L		Noodles	100
Lady fingers (10 cookies)	360		
Lamb (2 small chops)	250	**O**	
Lamb (leg of)	210	Oatmeal (1 cup cooked)	75
Lard (½ cup)	990	Oil (Codliver—1 tablespoon)	100
Leeks (3 medium)	40	Oil (Olive—1 tablespoon)	110
Lemon (1 medium)	20	Oil (Peanut—1 tablespoon)	125
Lentils	100	Oil (Salad—1 tablespoon)	125
Lettuce	20	Olives (6 small ones)	50
Lima beans (fresh or canned)	100	Onions (fresh—1 medium)	50
Lobster (boiled ¾ lb.)	90	Orange (average size)	75
Lobster (canned)	105	Orange juice (small glass)	65
Lobster (broiled—1 average)	300	Orange soda	75
		Oysters (12)	120
M			
Macaroni (cooked—1 cup)	155	**P**	
Macaroons	420	Parsley (1 tablespoon chopped)	1
Mackerel (broiled—3 oz.)	200	Parsnips (cooked)	45
Malaga (3 oz.)	120	Partridge	120
Malted milk powder (1 tbs.)	50	Pastry (1 average)	250
Manhattan (1 cocktail)	200	Pâté de foie gras	430
Margarine (1 oz.)	200	Peach (1 medium)	35
Marlin	80	Peach (canned, in syrup)	80
Marmalade (1 tablespoon)	50	Peach melba	375

Peach pie (1 slice)	375
Peanuts	670
Peanut butter (1 tablespoon)	90
Pear (1 medium)	95
Pear (canned, in syrup)	80
Pear pie (1 slice)	350
Peas (green—canned)	75
Peas (green—dried)	340
Pepper (1 medium)	20
Perch	90
Pheasant (roasted)	110
Pigeon	130
Pike	80
Pineapple (canned— 1 slice, syrup)	80
Pineapple (fresh—1 slice)	40
Pineapple juice (1 small glass)	70
Pistachio nuts (30)	90
Plum pudding (1 serving)	225
Plums (3 fresh green)	100
Plums (2 fresh red)	60
Pomegranate (1 medium)	80
Pork:	
Baked ham	450
Fillet of pork	195
Fresh pork	320
Pigs feet, pickled	230
Pork liver	150
Roast tenderloin	300
Roast pork	370
Salted pork	300
Port (3 oz.)	150
Potato (baked) unpeeled	100
Potato (boiled—1 medium)	100
Potato chips (10)	110
Potatoes (french-fried)	310
Potatoes (mashed)	120
Prunes (4 canned)	240
Prune juice (1 small glass)	85
Pumpkin	35

Q

Quail (1 broiled)	145
Quince (1 medium)	35

R

Rabbit (roasted—lean)	150
Rabbit (roasted—fatty)	220
Radishes (7)	15

Raisins	330
Raspberries	70
Raspberry pie (1 slice)	325
Red mullet	80
Rhubarb (fresh—1 cup diced)	20
Rum (1 oz.)	100
Rutabaga	35
Ry-Krisp (1)	15

S

Salami (¼-inch slice)	130
Salmon (canned—3 oz.)	175
Salmon (creamed)	200
Salmon (broiled—1 steak)	205
Salmon (smoked—3 oz.)	285
Salsify	75
Sandwich (average)	350
Sardines (canned, drained— 3 oz.)	180
Sauerkraut	15
Scallops	90
Semolina	360
Shad	190
Shrimp (fresh, 8 to 12)	125
Smelt (2 small)	50
Snails	75
Sole	80
Sole with butter (1 portion)	200
Sorrel	5
Soups: (1 cup)	
Asparagus, cream	200
Beef bouillon	10
Celery, cream	200
Chicken broth	50
Chicken, cream	200
Fish soup	90
Lentil	130
Mushroom, cream	200
Onion, clear	65
Split pea	200
Tomato broth	90
Tomato, cream	175
Vegetable	80
Spice cake (1 slice)	350
Spinach (cooked & seasoned)	25
Spinach (raw)	20
Squash, summer	15
Squash, winter (baked, mashed)	45

Strawberries (fresh)	45	Stew meat, (cooked—3 oz.)	250
Strawberry pie (1 slice)	300	Venison	110
Sturgeon (fresh)	120	Vienna sausage	250
Sugar (granulated)	440	Vinegar	0
Sweet potato (1 baked)	155	Vinaigrette sauce (1 tbs.)	20

T

Tangerine (1 medium)	40		
Tapioca pudding (½ cup)	150	**W**	
Tea (without sugar or milk)	0	Waffles (1 medium)	215
Toast, melba (1 slice)	25	Walnuts	325
Toast, white (1 slice)	65	Watercress (10 sprigs)	2
Tomato (1 medium)	30	Watermelon (1 slice)	120
Tongue (boiled—3 oz.)	205	Welsh rabbit (med. serving)	220
Trout, brook (broiled)	215	Whiskey: (per 1½ oz.)	
Trout, lake (broiled)	290	Bourbon	125
Truffles (fresh)	15	Rye	125
Tuna (canned, drained—3 oz.)	170	Scotch	115
Tuna (fresh—3 oz.)	150	White sauce (1 tablespoon)	25
Turkey, roasted	300	Wine, dry (3 oz.)	70
Turnips	20	Wine, sweet (3 oz.)	155
		Worcestershire sauce	
		(1 tablespoon)	10

V

Veal:

		Y	
Cutlet, breaded (1 medium)	215	Yoghurt	60
Roast, leg (1 medium size)	70		
Roast, shoulder (3 oz.)	190	**Z**	
		Zweibach toast (1 slice)	35